to my grandfather Judge Douglas Cameron (D.C.) Thomas and my stepfather, Professor John Tennyson (Jack) McLeod

Contents

Acknowledgements

I should like to thank my family for their constant support over the years, particularly my dear wife Janell, who patiently endured my research trips, formatted charts, and provided consistent encouragement. Thanks to my stepfather John Tennyson (Jack) McLeod, my mother Cynthia, my sister Adrienne, and my dear grandparents Douglas Cameron (D.C.) Thomas and Margaret (Arla) MacKay Thomas (dec.). I also thank the entire Harvey and Barounes clans for their warmth and support, particularly Maria and Gerry Harvey, and Edna Barounes (dec.). Thanks to Christina Greenough for her work on the index.

Thanks to my wonderful colleagues at The Colorado College for their friendship, intellectual camaraderie, and occasional critiques. My gratitude to Dr. Heinz Geppert for his assistance in translating several documents from archaic German. I should also like to thank Steve Tauber, Johnathan Daly, and Mark Amen of the University of South Florida, who provided valuable intellectual engagement and friendship during my early years in Florida.

Further, I owe a great debt to Steve Morse of the Mailman School of Public Health at Columbia University. Steve was instrumental in bringing me to Columbia for my post-doctoral work, and in my occasional returns since those early days. He has been profoundly influential in his support of the health and security debate, and in fostering global cooperation to prepare for emerging disease threats. Insight and encouragement was also provided by Daniel Deudney of the Department of Political Science at Johns Hopkins University. Dan's brave intellectual forays into republican theory provided a significant impetus to my work in recent years. I should also like to note the persistent intellectual influence of my doctoral advisor David A. Welch, and also that of Louis Pauly, Franklyn Griffiths, Salim Mansur, and Mark Zacher.

The research for this volume was supported by various grants and awards over the years. Generous patrons of this work include the Social Science Executive Committee, the Dean's Office at The Colorado College, the Christian-Johnson Foundation, the Benezet Award, the Mrachek Award, Asian Studies, and all of The Colorado College. Additional support was provided by the Center for Globalization of the University of South Florida, the US Department of Homeland Security, the US Department of Defense, and the World Affairs Councils of the United States. Finally I should like to thank my research assistants, Carmen Huckel, Rachel Shaffer, and Carlie Armstrong. I am grateful for the kind assistance I received from the library staff at the Statsbiobliothek Berlin, and at the Osterreichische Nationalbibliothek in Vienna. Finally, I should like to express my appreciation for the patience and diligence of my editors, Clay Morgan and Paul Bethge, and to the entire staff of the MIT Press.

Contagion and Chaos

Introduction

Great catastrophes may not necessarily give birth to genuine revolutions, but they infallibly herald them and make it necessary to think, or rather to think afresh, about the universe.
—Fernand Braudel (1980)

Health is the fulcrum of material power, and therefore it is central to the interests of the modern sovereign state. In the present day, novel trans-national threats to the security of states have arisen in the form of multinational terrorism, the proliferation of weapons of mass destruction, and global environmental change. From the mid 1990s on, scholars of international politics have speculated that emerging and re-emerging infectious diseases may also constitute a threat to international security, through their negative effects on sovereign states. Population health contributes directly to the endogenous prosperity and stability of a particular polity, to the consolidation and projection of sovereign power, and ultimately to the security of the state. The health of the body politic thus contributes directly to the functionality of the apparatus of governance.

Liberating the people from the shackles of disease and hunger contributes directly to the development and consolidation of endogenous human capital, which consequently augments economic productivity and the production of both social and technical ingenuity. The resulting prosperity permits the extraction of fiscal resources from the people via mechanisms of taxation to fill the coffers of the state. In view of the fungibility of economic power, such revenues may be transformed into public goods delivered to the people, or channeled into the apparatus of coercion (the military and police) so as to maintain order and project power abroad.

The antithesis of health, epidemic disease, then, presents a direct threat to the power of the state, as it erodes prosperity, destabilizing the relations between state and society, renders institutions sclerotic, foments intra-state violence, and ultimately diminishes the power and cohesion of the state. As such, epidemic infectious disease is profoundly disruptive to an affected polity, undermining its security. Yet contagion also contains the seeds of catalytic socio-economic and political transformation.

The principle of creative destruction lies at the core of all natural processes of change.[1] Geologists speak of catastrophic disruptions produced by phenomena such as volcanism, earthquakes, and impact events, yet out of such chaotic periods a new order emerges. Fire sweeps through an ecosystem, devastating the local flora and fauna, and in the aftermath a new ecological equilibrium coalesces. In these natural processes one sees a pattern: an original period of stasis and equilibrium, then a period of chaotic destabilization (turbulence), and then the establishment of a second equilibrium that may differ radically from the one that preceded the destruction. Thus, natural systems exhibit periods of stasis followed by abrupt change—a model of punctuated equilibrium, if you will.[2] The human species (and the institutions it has fashioned) emerged in the context of such catalytic (and non-linear) processes, and despite our anthropocentric hubris we remain deeply embedded within the global ecology, subject to droughts, hurricanes, earthquakes, and epidemic diseases.

Historians have argued that contagion wrought profound changes in the socio-economic, legal, and political orders of afflicted societies.[3] Yet the complex interplay between non-linear natural systems and human societies is often ignored within the social sciences, particularly in the domain of political science.[4] The political scientist Daniel Deudney has deplored the lack of inclusion of material-contextual factors in present-day political science, which acts as if societies evolved and matured *ex nihilo*: "[A] major distorting filter in contemporary thinking, particularly about international relations . . . is a gross underappreciation or misappreciation of the importance of material-contextual factors, of nature, geography, ecology, and technology. We think and act as if technologies are just our handy tools and as if nature has somehow just been left behind."[5]

Historians have continued to investigate how such material-contextual variables (including contagion) affect state-society relations. Fernand

Braudel, one of the foremost historians of the twentieth century, noted that manifestations of epidemic disease induced profound disruptions of existing institutions such as markets, economies, and socio-political systems, and that such disruptions could be protracted.[6] In a Schumpeterian sense, epidemics have the capacity to induce profound turmoil but often function as catalysts of change, generating transformation in the belief structures of survivors, in the micro- and macro-level social and economic structures of affected polities, in the relations between the state and society, and ultimately between countries. The profoundly destabilizing effects of contagion result from various manifestations of illness, including high levels of mortality and/or morbidity, the destruction of human capital, economic disruption, negative psychological effects, the consequent acrimony between affected social factions, and the deteriorating relations between the people and an often draconian state.

The reader will, doubtless, note the double-entendre in the title of this book. The historical record suggests that contagion may induce degrees of chaos within affected societies, the level being dependent on many subtle contextual variables regarding the pathogen, the affected society, and the resilience (or capacity) of the state. In addition, the emergence of novel pathogenic microbial agents results from the complex interplay of chaotic systems in the natural realm, and from their intersection with the human ecology. Natural systems exhibit non-linearities (such as epidemic growth curves) and emergent properties, govern the emergence of novel zoonoses, and determine the course of their manifestation as epidemic and/or pandemic disease. Such non-linear dynamics are often observed during periods of war. To the extent that war destroys the infrastructure of medicine, public health, and sanitation, impedes the production and distribution of food and medical supplies, prevents surveillance and treatment, and generates poverty, it is a driver of pathogenic emergence and virulence. To that end, the social and structural chaos induced by war may act as a powerful amplifier of disease.[7]

Hypotheses

The first hypothesis advanced in this volume is that epidemic disease may function as a stressor variable to compromise the prosperity, the legitimacy, the structural cohesion, and in certain cases the security of sovereign states. Further, disease may exacerbate pre-existing domestic conflicts between ethnicities, and/or classes and may generate intra-societal and intra-state violence, and the resulting societal discord may generate punitive and draconian responses by the state against the people as it seeks to maintain order. Thus, disease often functions to destabilize the coherence, the power, and (perhaps) the security of the state.

The second hypothesis is that epidemic and pandemic manifestations of novel pathogens may promote economic and political discord between countries, although contagion is not likely to generate significant armed conflict between sovereign states.

The third hypothesis is that only some of the documented infectious pathogens threaten national security, and that criteria based on lethality, transmissibility, fear, and economic damage will illuminate which pathogens are security threats and which are not.

The fourth hypothesis is that the practices of warfare (both intra-state and inter-state) will generate "war pestilences," contributing to the proliferation of infectious disease within the ranks of the combatants and subsequently to proximate civilian populations. Thus, conflict amplifies the burden of disease.

The fifth hypothesis is that the paradigm of "health security" is philosophically grounded in the political tradition of republican theory, a theoretical antecedent to both Realism and Liberalism; that the association between the health of the population and perceptions of national security is ancient but largely forgotten; and that a republican revision of systems-level international relations theory (with elements of political psychology) provides an optimal theoretical framework for pursuing such inquiries.

The biologist E. O. Wilson bemoaned the "fragmentation of knowledge" and argued that the solutions to the complex collective action problems of the modern age lay in interdisciplinary knowledge and its practical application. This volume is explicitly a consilient,[8] or interdisciplinary, exploration of the relationship among infectious disease, governance, and prosperity within affected polities, and between countries. The material presented herein is admittedly an eclectic synthesis of political science, history, biology, demography, economics, psychology, sociology, ecology, physics, and public health. The hope is that such a work may appeal to a broad audience and encourage new avenues of thought and investigation across the disciplines, bridging the epistemic schisms that have deepened over the decades as a result of disciplinary specialization.

On Globalization and Disease

A considerable amount of scholarly discourse has emerged concerning the effect of globalization on economies and societies, but such literature typically ignores the nexus of globalization, ecology, and public health. Processes of "globalization"[9] are often linked to the diffusion of pathogens in the modern era, as trade is directly associated with the inter-continental diffusion of pathogens and with their vectors of transmission.[10] Global microbial proliferation and emergence is also facilitated by tourism and migration, by increasing population densities, by environmental degradation,[11] by international (and intra-state) conflict,[12] and (to a degree) by inequities in the international distribution of resources between developed and developing countries.[13] Thus, the proliferation of pathogenic organisms is a negative manifestation of globalization, but such processes are by no means novel, although the scale and rapidity of emergence has increased.

The emergence and diffusion of infectious disease on a global scale is a process that originated during the earliest years of inter-continental trade. The first recorded instance of such trade-induced pathogenic diffusion was the "plague" of Athens, which was borne to Greece by trade ships from Northern Africa.[14] In the centuries that followed, plague bacilli (*Yersinia pestis*) came to Europe via trade caravans from Central Asia along the Silk Road,[15] and Europeans transmitted the scourge of smallpox to Native American populations with the "discovery" of the Americas.[16] In recent decades we have witnessed profound qualitative changes in the processes of globalization (e.g., the rapidly increased speed of trade and migration as facilitated by advances in transportation technologies, which augments the speed and scale of pathogenic proliferation). Furthermore, the diffusion of both knowledge and fear via telecommunications media permit the negative psychological externalities produced by disease to affect the global community, as was demonstrated by the SARS[17] epidemic of 2003. Furthermore, globalization may accelerate the evolutionary properties of pathogens, augmenting their natural disposition to swap genetic information. William Rosen notes that globalization has increased the genetic "library of code"[18] available to all microorganisms as pathogens from disparate and previously isolated regions have become able to exchange genetic properties with other ubiquitous organisms. Further, the burgeoning human population increases the sheer number of organisms in the human ecology, and the increasing speed of travel accelerates the global process of genetic mixing.

The Scope of the Problem

During the Cold War (1945–1991), issues of public health (with the exception of biological weaponry) were typically consigned to the realm of "low politics." With the end of US-Soviet rivalry in the early 1990s, environmental change, terrorism, migration, and public health began to ascend on the international agenda. Public health victories against microbes reached a zenith in the mid 1970s with the development of powerful anti-microbial drugs. However, the pace and intensity of pathogen emergence has increased since that time with the proliferation of novel agents of contagion. In the late 1990s, the recognition that the HIV/AIDS pandemic represented a significant threat to the economy, the governance, and perhaps the security of developing countries spurred the academic and policy communities into action against this emerging foe. In recent years, the BSE epizootic, the SARS contagion of 2003, and our increasing understanding of the influenza pandemic of 1918–19 have generated great interest in the political and economic impact of contagion. Such outcomes include a capacity to generate socio-political acrimony, a capacity to disrupt global markets and trade, and a capacity to disrupt relations within and between sovereign states.

The Modern Literature on Public Health and Security

Over the centuries, various schools of thought have emerged to examine the linkages between public health and governance. Historians have long dominated the debate, beginning with Thucydides. In recent times, Alfred Crosby, William McNeill, and Peter Baldwin have argued that interactions between pathogens and the human ecology often generate profound effects on the evolutionary trajectories of human societies. In the domain of political science, the first inquiries into the relationship among public health, governance, and security were articulated by Dennis Pirages (1995), who argued for the emerging concept of "microsecurity" and pushed for a re-conceptualization of security to include non-military threats.[19] Pirages was followed by other political scientists, including Price-Smith (1999, 2001), Elbe (2002), Ostergard (2002, 2007), Peterson (2002, 2006), Singer (2002), Huang (2003), Youde (2005), and McInnes (2006). In the realm of public health and international law, the legal scholars David Fidler (1999) and Obi Aginam (2005) have conducted inquiries into the nature and depth of cooperation between sovereign entities and international organizations, often crossing over into political science. Collectively, the work of this group constitutes the discourse that forms the canon of the "health security" debate in the domain of political science.

Plan of the Book

In chapter 1, I offer a historical exploration of relations between state and society in the context of contagion, ranging from Thucydides' observations to relatively recent times. The purpose here is to expose the reader to the utility of the historical record as a means to inform modern inquiries in the social sciences. Disease has historically generated negative effects on various societies, ranging from economic and social destabilization to rampant stigmatization and inter-ethnic violence, prompting draconian reactions by the state against its own people to enforce order. In that chapter I also illustrate the principle that infectious disease has long been perceived as a distinct threat to stability, to prosperity, to the material interests of elite factions, and therefore to the security of the state. This serves to place the current debate as to whether disease should be "securitized" in its proper historical perspective.

In chapter 2, I analyze the effects of the influenza pandemic of 1918–19 on various affected societies. In the domain of demography, the chapter illustrates the differential mortality generated by the waves of contagion that swept the planet. The chapter then examines the possibility that the pandemic affected the various combatants in World War I in different fashions, based on the statistical data presented herein. Previously unpublished data from German and Austrian archives reveal the malign effects of the virus on the military forces and the people of the Central Powers during this period. Analysis of the data suggests that the epidemic eroded the Central Powers' capacity to continue the conflict, and that it may have accelerated their capitulation and/or disintegration. The data presented herein also raise the possibility that the first serious episode of influenza-induced mortality occurred in Austria in the spring of 1917, not in the United States in the spring of 1918. Finally, the chapter briefly addresses the Swine Flu affair and the shortcomings of the United States' preparedness for another lethal pandemic.

Chapter 3 constitutes an analysis of the deleterious effects of HIV/AIDS on intra-societal relations, the capacity of state institutions, and the relations of the state to society in the context of the contagion. In that chapter I examine the worst-case scenario of Zimbabwe and juxtapose it against the scenario of Botswana, where, despite similarly high levels of contagion, state-society relations remain benign and the state retains its cohesion. The chapter examines the demographic implications of HIV/AIDS, and in particular the issue of AIDS orphans and their potential for radicalization. Using a human-capital approach, I then analyze the effects of HIV/AIDS on economic productivity (at the micro, sectoral, and macro levels) and the virus' possible effects on foreign investment. Subsequently, I examine the effects of the pathogen on the domain of governance, articulating the direct negative effects of HIV/AIDS on the institutions of the state, such as the military, police forces, and the bureaucracy. Finally, I chronicle the Zimbabwe government's draconian response and abuses of power, which have coincided with the epidemic, and collectively undermined societal prosperity and cohesion.

Chapter 4 is an investigation into the effects of a prion-induced contagion, bovine spongiform encephalopathy (BSE), and its human variant, Creutzfeld-Jakob disease. In both Europe and North America, the BSE affair is associated with questions about the efficacy and legitimacy of the scientific community and about the government institutions that are entrusted with safeguarding the public interest. In this chapter I also analyze the economic impact of these cases and explore how the North American cases generated externalities that continue to undermine the United States' relations with Japan and South Korea. I highlight problems of miscalculation of risk, question assumptions of rationality by individuals and states, and note the significant role of emotion (fear and anxiety). Further, I examine the role of BSE in generating rapid institutional change at both the domestic and the international level, and I analyze BSE's effects on cooperation between sovereign states.

In chapter 5 I deal with the SARS contagion of 2002–03, which resulted from the emergence of a novel coronavirus in southern China late in the year 2002. I detail the peculiar etiology of the virus and its subsequent demographic impact. I also note the central role of fear and anxiety in undermining social cohesion, international markets, and the irrational behavior of many sovereign states in the face of a new pathogen. I then examine the effects of SARS on governance in China and Canada, and on regional governance in Pacific Rim countries. Finally, I examine the claim that we have entered a "post-Westphalian" era of global health governance.

In chapter 6, I analyze violent conflict and war as "disease amplifiers." I examine the mechanisms by which inter-state and intra-state conflict contribute to the dissemination of existing pathogens and to the emergence of novel microbial agents. I then examine the interaction between conflict and individual pathogens as documented in the historical record. I utilize data regarding the incidence of multiple pathogens and their effects on mortality and morbidity culled from US, German, and Austrian government archives for the period of World War I (1914–1918), and the role of civil wars in the propagation of disease.

In chapter 7, I briefly examine the proposition that health contributes to economic productivity, which then bolsters the power of the state and facilitates the projection of power (martial and ideological). I chronicle the nascent debate on health security and critique the existing literature. I then argue that significant pathogenic threats to health constitute both a direct and an indirect threat to national security. Further, I argue that the existing "health and security" debate is excessively myopic, insofar as most of the current discourse focuses exclusively on HIV/AIDS, and that as a result the discourse is profoundly anti-historical. Moreover, this debate in political science reveals a truncated understanding of the history of public health, and of health's effects on state-society relations. Finally, I suggest a mechanism by which security theorists may assess the threat that a specific pathogen presents to a specific state.

1

Theory and Exegesis: On Health and the Body Politic

Most of the change we think we see in life
Is due to truths being in and out of favor
—Robert Frost, "The Black Cottage"

My analysis does not seek to explain all possible outcomes related to the effects of disease on structures of governance, but rather to generate plausible analytical relationships between variables that will permit further empirical testing and refinement. As the philosopher of science Thomas Kuhn stated, "To be accepted as a paradigm, a theory must seem better than its competitors, but it need not, and in fact never does, explain all the facts with which it can be confronted."[1]

On *Physis* and Republican Theory

In *The Social Contract*, the Swiss republican political philosopher Jean-Jacques Rousseau explicitly linked population health, economic productivity, and effective governance:

What is the object of any political association? It is the protection and prosperity of its members. And what is the surest evidence that they are so protected and prosperous? The numbers of their population. Then do not look beyond this much debated evidence. All other things being equal, the government under which, without external aids . . . the citizens increase and multiply most is infallibly the best government. That under which the people diminishes and wastes away is the worst.[2]

Indeed, Rousseau recognized that implementation of the social contract effectively entailed an exchange between the sovereign and the governed wherein the latter pledged their fealty (and taxes) to the former in exchange for the protection of their lives and property: "Their very lives which they have pledged to the state, are always protected by it. . . ."[3] Such duties of the state were noted by the English republican political theorist Thomas Hobbes, who argued in *Leviathan* that the state possessed a fundamental obligation to protect its people from predation by external agents (i.e., foreign militaries) or by internal agents (criminals).[4] One might certainly extend the argument to posit that the state is also obligated to protect the people from pathogenic forms of predation. States that fail to protect their citizens from predation may be viewed as in violation of the social contract. Such failures erode governmental claims to legitimacy in the eyes of the much diminished and debilitated people. In the domain of the political, both Rousseau and Hobbes are claimed as part of the Realist tradition, yet, as Daniel Deudney and Nicholas Onuf argue, they are in fact best conceived of as belonging to an antecedent and "republican" tradition of political thought. Realpolitik and Liberalism, which originated in the nineteenth century, then are conceptualized as the analytical descendants of this earlier republican school, and facets of both of these successor paradigms may be located in that earlier theoretical progenitor.[5]

To provide conceptual clarity, I adopt Deudney's concise definition of a republic as "a political order marked by political freedom, popular sovereignty, and limited government."[6] The republican tradition, which was certainly dominant in ancient Greek thought (Aristotle, Plato, Thucydides), was based in part on Aristotle's heralded debate between *physis* (nature) and *nomos* (convention) and the mutual influence they exerted upon each other.[7] Ultimately, Aristotle held that *physis* provided the basis for the emergence of *nomos*, and thus the natural world profoundly influences the derivative world of human constructs, such as political entities.[8] Aristotle was therefore the progenitor of structural-materialist thought in political philosophy. Plato concurred, and argued that *physis* constituted a powerful driver of political transformation. Such logic was particularly evident in his chronicling of various natural disasters (earthquakes, floods, fires) that devastated human societies and left the survivors to reconstruct (or re-invent) their modes of social and political association.[9]

The Hellenic republican tradition infused Western political thought and informed Machiavelli, Rousseau, Montesquieu, and Hobbes, who also held that material-contextual variables[10] were of profound significance in determining the trajectory of political affairs, both domestically and internationally.[11]

Such material factors were often cast as forces of "nature" and regarded as representing constraints and/or opportunities for a polity.[12] Montesquieu also noted the pivotal role of *physis* when he proclaimed that "the empire of climate is the first and most powerful of empires."[13] This is certainly logical from an epidemiological perspective, insofar as the disease gradient and the aggregate burden of disease on a society increase dramatically as one moves from temperate climes into the tropics. As Deudney argues, Montesquieu's work is central to understanding the relations between *physis* and *polis*, and Montesquieu stands as a pivotal empiricist in the domain of political thought even though much of modern international relations theory ignores his work. "Montesquieu's materialist arguments," Deudney writes, "are marshaled as part of a general effort to explain the origins and differences in the mores and laws of particular societies."[14]

In the post–Cold War era, the rise of environmental politics, and the environment-and-security debate in particular, sought to resurrect the decisive role of *physis* with some partial success,[15] although political science in the early twenty-first century maintains its profoundly ideational bias. In his exemplary discussion of the role of *physis* in republican discourse, Deudney argues that "the physical world is not completely or primarily subject to effective human control and . . . natural material-contextual realities impede or enable vital and recurring human goals. Such arguments attempt to link specific physical constraints and opportunities given by nature to alterations in the performance of very basic functional tasks universal to human groups."[16] Leo Strauss echoed this axiom of the fundamental role of *physis*, and the Aristotelian search for "first causes," when he argued that "the discovery of nature is the work of philosophy."[17]

Thus, Realist theory is heir to the materialist tradition of republican theory, particularly in its application of technological change to questions of security (e.g., the development of nuclear weapons).[18] Realists seek to explain politics as it is, and not as it ought to be, suggesting that there are fixed and empirically based laws that govern the political sphere. Conversely, the poverty of much "critical" or post-modern political theory emanates from its blatant omission of material-contextual factors, including demography, geography, energy, advances in technology, and the subject of this discourse, population health.[19] Largely as a consequence of Weberian thought, political discourse in the late twentieth century exhibited the increasing dominance of the ideational over the material, impoverishing current debates. The extreme marginalization of material variables within the predominant political discourse is problematic, as it leads to the inaccurate assumption that human societies are no longer subject to the laws of nature (and thus completely divorced from *physis*). Conversely, an extension of Aristotelian logic would hold that material-contextual factors are primal and intrinsically important, and that they form the empirical basis for ideational variables such as culture, identity, and political constructs. Of course, this relationship between physis and nomos exhibits evidence of reciprocal causation, as human society (largely through technological ingenuity) has over the centuries increasingly altered nature through its actions.

Such material-contextual factors continue to operate at both the domestic (or unit) level and the international (or system) level, freeing us of the dichotomization of modern political analysis into the domestic and system levels of analysis. While such divisions may suit intellectuals who seek parsimony, they are profoundly incapable of dealing with the many trans-boundary issues that now vex human societies. For example, emergent and re-emergent pathogens (e.g., SARS and HIV) originate within states, often function as global collective action problems, and ignore the porous political boundaries of sovereign states. In the same vein, environmental collective action problems (e.g., protection of the atmospheric and oceanic commons) routinely cross the unit/system level boundary. Onuf argues that this division itself is a legacy of Weberian thought, notably its second modern phase: ". . . social thought and practice before modernity's second phase . . . made no clear distinction between social relations within and among states."[20]

In this analytical domain, republican theory diverges from its theoretical successors, as both Realist and Liberal theories presuppose a sharp delineation between international and domestic politics, the latter having little if any influence on conduct between polities in the former. However, the empirical reality is that many problems arising within the territory of a sovereign state may defy containment within that polity, and function as externalities that destabilize not only contiguous countries but also (in some cases) distant polities and/or the entire international system. For example, an infectious disease arising in China (e.g., SARS) may not remain contained within that polity but may proliferate throughout East Asia and North America, and may destabilize global economic relations. In similar fashion, failed states generate externalities that often affect the entire system, as did the rise of Al-Qaeda under the

Taliban in the failed state of Afghanistan. The political scientist James Rosenau echoes this skepticism toward the unit/system level dichotomization, holding that "in a rapidly changing, interdependent world the separation of national and international affairs is problematic."[21] Rosenau argues that this porous and nebulous domain of interaction between the domestic and international levels is best conceptualized as "the Frontier."

Another area of divergence between republican theory and orthodox late-twentieth-century Realism lies in the latter's almost exclusive focus on relations between the great powers, and the general neglect of middle powers and smaller states as "inconsequential" to the operations and mechanics of the global system. In the realm of infectious disease, however, global pathogenic threats may emanate from failed states or quasi-states, or from those polities that exhibit low endogenous capacity, with poor public health infrastructure, entrenched poverty and structural inequities, high population density, and ecological degradation.[22] Thus, owing to dynamics of global interdependence, processes at work within the weakest countries on the planet may generate negative externalities that ultimately compromise the material interests, and perhaps even the national security, of the great powers. This emphasis on complex interdependence between sovereign countries, particularly in the realm of trans-national issues, is the domain of republican theory's other successor, Liberalism. Yet the notion that disease could be transferred from one society to another is ancient, finding its first manifestations in Thucydides' account of the Plague of Athens, which suggests that the plague was imported via trade from Africa.[23]

As Rousseau noted, the health and size of a given population would certainly have been regarded as indispensable to the vitality of that body politic, and to the puissance of that nation. The manifestation of pathogenic infectious disease represented (and represents) a direct threat to the population base, erodes economic productivity, often weakens the institutions of the state and its ability to provide public goods, compromises governmental legitimacy, and often led to intra-class and/or intra-ethnic conflict within the state. Thus, an exogenous agent could act to fundamentally threaten the material interests and the stability of the affected polity in question. Furthermore, republican theory is concerned with placing constraints on the development of hierarchy within the state, recognizing the potential for despotic government and violence, directed by the state against its own people. Such concerns become readily apparent in the chapters that follow as the disruptions induced by plague, cholera, HIV, and pandemic influenza often resulted in draconian violence by the state against the people in order to quell the disruption engendered by the pathogen in question.

It is not the purpose of this volume to reconstruct international relations theory. However, I should like to make a few brief observations, and I recommend a republican revision of Realist theory. Such a revision entails maintaining certain postulates of Realism, that the international system is anarchical, that this state of anarchy is primarily competitive, and that sovereign states remain the dominant actors in international politics. Moreover, Realist theory states that states seek to maximize their power in order to attain their primary goal of survival. A republican revision entails considerable modification to Realist orthodoxy. First, echoing the work of the political scientist Robert Jervis, republican Realism abandons assumptions of the Rational Actor Model, holding that foreign policy is often driven by powerful elites and factions within the state, and that these policy makers are subject to cognitive and affective limitations. Thus human nature, human limitations and their effects upon rational decision-making are brought back into Realist theory.[24] Furthermore, republican theory eschews orthodox Realism's fixation upon great power politics as ethnocentric, and holds that interactions between all states (including middle and small powers) are worthy of analysis. Moreover, while states remain the central actors in international politics, republican models accept the rise of non-state actors and other challenges (environmental degradation, disease) as threats to the material interests (and security) of sovereign states. Finally, a republican revision of Realism notes that the harsh dichotomization between the system and domestic levels of analysis is analytically problematic, particularly given that diseases, environmental degradation, or radical networks within a given state may generate externalities that compromise proximate states, and perhaps affect the system in its entirety.

A central claim of the present work is that pathogens can act as stressors on societies, economies, and institutions of governance. The proliferation of infectious disease may thereby compromise state capacity, and may destabilize the institutional architecture of the state. Under certain conditions, infectious disease may therefore represent a direct and/or an indirect threat to the material interests of the state, and therefore to national security. Thus, I pursue a state-centric theory of analysis, but one that acknowledges the complex interaction between state and society

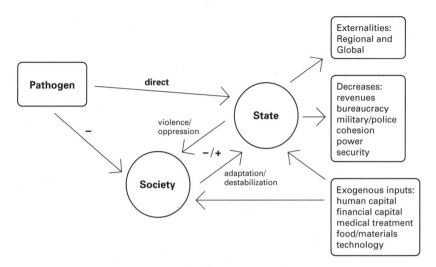

Figure 1.1
Theoretical construct of possible relations.

in the context of contagion. (See figure 1.1.) This conceptualization of the relations between variables—an extension of previous work (Price-Smith 2001)—includes significant revisions to the original model: society is included as an intervening variable, and it is specified that effects on the dependent variable (state capacity) can generate radiating externalities that affect entire geographic regions and possibly the global system.

The Independent Variable: Pathogens

Emergent or re-emergent pathogens constitute the independent variable. They are, by definition, novel and autonomous empirical agents that have recently become endogenized (or re-endogenized) within the human ecology. The etiology, the lethality, and the vectors of transmission of an emergent pathogen are initially obscure, and therefore the agent may generate enormous uncertainty, anxiety, and fear in affected populations. Re-emerging infections include those pathogens that are becoming re-established in human populations where they had formerly been minimized or eradicated, such that the human population no longer possesses substantial levels of acquired immunity to ward off the contagion. While the historical effects of diverse pathogens are explored in the next chapter, the case studies that follow focus on four emergent pathogens in the post-1900 era (pandemic influenza, HIV, the SARS coronavirus, and the BSE prion) in order to investigate whether the historical effects of contagion on the state and society (and on their interface) remain potent and malign.

The Intervening Variable: Society

Virulent and destructive pathogens may affect the state directly, or their effects on the state may be mediated through the intervening variable of society. The Oxford English Dictionary defines a society as "the aggregate of people living together in a more or less ordered community [and] a particular community of people living in a country or region, and having shared customs, laws, and organizations." Factions or interest groups within society are linked together through social networks, or what the sociologist Robert Putnam has called "social capital."[25] Further, societies exhibit an enormous degree of variation in belief structures, in norms, and particularly in degree of complexity.[26] Society may, therefore, exacerbate the destabilizing effects of the pathogen on the state as it disintegrates into rival factions based on class or ethnicity, or it may generate successful adaptive strategies to ameliorate the effects of contagion.

Contagion may affect society in diverse fashions, as pathogen-induced effects in one domain (e.g., economics) radiate to generate pernicious outcomes in another (e.g., the political). In the domain of demography, pathogens will induce varying degrees of morbidity and mortality of the population, may affect fertility, and may induce emigration from affected regions. In the domain of economics, pathogens will compromise the productivity of workers[27] and may impose a range of direct and indirect costs on firms, families, sectors, and the macro economy. Further, contagion may destabilize markets through supply-and-demand-induced shocks, erode domestic savings, affect patterns of foreign investment into afflicted countries, and inhibit macro-level economic productivity.[28] Disease-induced economic contraction may also result in diminished revenues for the state through taxation, inhibiting its capacity to deliver public services, reducing its legitimacy, and compromising its security relative to foreign rivals. In the domain of psychology, contagion may generate significant negative effects, such as increasing uncertainty, suboptimal risk assessment, misperception, significant levels of affect (emotion), the construction of images of self and other, and the stigmatization of the ill. Pernicious outcomes in these domains may combine to undermine social networks, compromise societal cohesion, undermine societal resilience, and even generate violence between ethnic groups or between classes. The political scientist Joel Migdal has noted that exogenous shocks (including outbreaks of epidemic disease) can induce significant social destabilization and can affect relations between state and society: "Natural disaster, war, and other extraordinary circumstances can greatly decrease the overall level of social control in societies by taking rewards and sanctions out of the hands of leaders of social organizations or by making the strategies of survival they offer irrelevant to the new exigencies people face."[29]

The Dependent Variable: The State

Pathogenic effects on the capacity of the state may be either indirect (mediated by society) or direct, whereupon contagion may result in the debilitation or destruction of the state's human assets (soldiers, police, bureaucrats) and in the weakening of state institutions. The state is defined as "an organization, composed of numerous agencies led and coordinated by the state's leadership (executive authority) that has the ability or authority to make and implement the binding rules for all the people as well as the parameters of rule making for other social organizations in a given territory, using force if necessary to have its way."[30] State capacity, then, refers to the power, capability, and autonomy of the state, and therefore indicates the capability of government.[31] Capacity is composed of various components, including fiscal resources, resilience, legitimacy, reach and responsiveness, coherence, autonomy, human capital, and coercive power (both internal and external). Moreover, capacity determines the state's ability to maximize its prosperity, stability, and projection of power, to exert *de facto* and *de jure* control over its territory, to protect its population from predation, and to adapt to diverse crises. "State capacity," then, refers to the endogenous capability of government, and its level determines the state's ability to satisfy its most important needs: survival, protection of its citizens from physical harm, economic prosperity and stability, effective governance, territorial integrity, power projection, and ideological projection.[32] In the case studies that follow, we will assess the impact of infectious disease (the independent variable) on state capacity in order to determine the possible pathways of associations between variables. This will allow us to construct robust qualitative hypotheses, which may facilitate further quantitative analyses in subsequent investigations.

Postulates

Previous inquiries suggest that the following postulates regarding the impact of contagion on society, the state, and relations between them may hold at the domestic level. Effects are delineated according to domain of inquiry, and then tested against the historical data and the pathogen-specific cases in the chapters that follow.

Domestic

Demographic Impacts   Infectious disease often results in significant negative outcomes for human health, ranging from debilitation to death. Possible outcomes include a sickened population, widespread mortality and contraction of the population, and the contraction of specific age cohorts within a population (as in the case of HIV/AIDS). Epidemics may also generate rapid and significant migration from affected areas as people attempt to flee the source of infection.

Psychological Impacts   The psychological repercussions of contagion typically include significant levels of emotion (notably fear and anxiety) that typically impede Pareto-optimal rationality in decision making at both the individual and the collective level. Such emotion is primarily a product of uncertainty and of inaccurate estimation of risk. Emotional and perceptual distortions may also generate the construction of images of the "other," resulting in stigmatization, persecution of minorities, and even diffuse inter-ethnic or inter-class violence. High levels of emotion combine with information that conflicts with individual belief structures to generate cognitive dissonance, wherein individuals engage in denial of the discrepant information in order to minimize psychological pain.

Economic Impacts   Disease-induced destruction/debilitation of the base of human capital erodes the productivity of workers, imposes direct and indirect costs on families, firms, and the state, depletes savings, and compromises a society's ability to generate social and technical ingenuity. At the macro level, disease generates a significant contraction in the production possibilities of a particular economy, perhaps even generating economic dislocation and decline in severe cases. Such contraction imposes constraints on the revenues that the state may extract from the people through taxation, further limiting its capacity. And if instability is perceived, infectious disease may undermine foreign investment in seriously affected regions.

Governance   Outbreaks of disease often shift power from the people to the state as the state increasingly imposes draconian controls in an attempt to contain the contagion, and/or to limit the socio-economic disruption associated with the outbreak of disease. Second, disease may generate competition and even conflict between classes or between elites, and may also manifest in the form of inter-ethnic conflict. Third, disease may generate a sclerotic effect on the apparatus of governance, wherein the state's capacity to deliver essential services becomes increasingly curtailed, impairing the government's legitimacy. Governments may become increasingly paralytic[33] as institutions become fragile and ineffective. Fourth, as social relations become increasingly chaotic, and as the state destabilizes, the state may engage in draconian and coercive practices against the population in order to maintain cohesion and order.

Externalities   Pathogen-induced destabilization at the domestic level may generate negative externalities that affect other states in the international system. Such unpalatable externalities may include economic destabilization, disruption of trade, migratory flows, and even political destabilization. Thus, analytical models must deal with high levels of interactivity and connectivity between agents and outcomes at the domestic and international levels.

International

Economic Impacts   The emergence, and subsequent proliferation of novel pathogens generates profound morbidity and mortality, uncertainty, and fear. Contagion may destabilize markets, may undercut international trade and commerce, and (if there is a quarantine) may limit the trans-national movement of both trade goods and personnel (i.e., human capital).

Governance Impacts   Contagion may foster political acrimony, may erode the effective function of international organizations, and may expose persistent problems in cooperation between sovereign states and other agents in the realm of global health governance. Contrary to earlier hypotheses in the health security literature, disease is unlikely to directly induce armed conflict between sovereign states. However, disease may compromise a state's ability to defend itself and, over a longer term, its ability to project power (martial, fiscal, and ideological).

Case Studies and Selection

Previous work in the field of health security has revealed negative empirical linkages between disease and state capacity,[34] and between disease and the incidence of intra-state violence.[35] However, it is prudent to re-examine the dominant hypotheses within the field and reconceptualize the relations among pathogens, society, and the state. Qualitative exploration of the probable relations among variables, through case studies that examine the interactivity of various domains (demographic, economic, social, psychological), may illuminate linkages that heretofore have remained obscure.[36] The case studies presented below analyze the effects of various pathogens on state-society dynamics to reveal historical patterns of behavior and reaction. The postulates developed from the available historical evidence may then be examined in the context of modern manifestations of contagion for the purpose of evaluating to what extent such historical patterns may still apply.

Thomas Kuhn offered a rationale for the case study/synthesis approach: "In the absence of a paradigm or some candidate for paradigm, all of the facts that could possibly pertain to the development of a given science are likely to seem equally relevant. As a result early fact-gathering is a far more nearly random activity than the one that subsequent scientific development makes familiar. . . . Early fact-gathering is usually restricted to the wealth of data that lie ready at hand."[37] Moreover, analyses that focus on a single variable, assuming that others will remain constant, are flawed, as changes in the primary variable may generate significant variance in the others.[38] Thus, even though infectious disease is the independent variable in each of our cases, it is inaccurate to assume that intervening variables (such as societal institutions) remain constant—they do not. The rationale underlying comparisons and case studies (as delineated by pathogen) is by no means novel. Indeed, the medical historian Charles Rosenberg explicitly argued for such a comparative approach based on his conceptualization of "the individuality of disease entities."[39] Pathogens will exhibit differential effects on polities according to lethality, mode of transmission, and psychological effects. Because of such complex systemic interactions, I will employ a series of case studies, selected according to pathogen, to examine the effects of contagion on state-society dynamics, state capacity, and inter-state relations. Each case study will analyze the impact of a particular pathogen on various domains (e.g., demography, psychology, economics, governance) and will then analyze the interactions among domains. The net result will be the generation of probable associations between variables that will permit refined empirical testing of hypotheses and will reduce the probability of spurious correlations or linkages that have no basis in public health or in medicine.

As criteria for selecting cases, I used the following:

· The case must analyze the effect of one specific pathogen.
· The pathogen must be emergent or re-emergent in that it was a novel agent in the twentieth century or thereafter.
· The pathogen must have generated at least some disruption (economic, social, or political) within the populations of five sovereign states.

The number of case studies (four) is admittedly small, but they are buttressed by a historical comparison of the effects of various pathogens on states and societies across millennia. Despite the small number of studies, the findings should permit preliminary generalizations about the probable relations among variables. The political scientist Steven Walt defends this approach, noting that increasing the number of case studies does not necessarily translate into increased analytical accuracy: "We are often better off with a small number of *valid* observations, as opposed to a large number of observations that do not really tap the concept that we are trying to explore."[40] Furthermore, statistical explorations typically assume linear relations among variables, and cannot easily deal with non-linear systems, feedback loops, thresholds, and multiple chains of causal interactions between variables. As such this analysis is conducted using methods of tracing processes across domains to reveal these complex and interactive relations.[41]

The case-study approach is propitious, as it illustrates the possible pathways of interaction between various agents and nodes within complex bio-political systems. Only through examination of the connectivity between domains (demographic, economic, psychological) at the domestic level can we illuminate pathogen-specific modes of interaction within a polity. Furthermore, the effects of contagion on state and society are often pathogen-specific, with certain agents generating profound negative psychological effects that compound the problems generated by mortality, morbidity, and economic dislocation. Thus, before we can engage in large-*N*, multi-variate statistical regressions that assume linear functions, we must know what we are looking for. Hence the need for the pathogen-specific case studies that examine the effect of a specific agent on the system.

Chaos, Non-Linearity, and Emergent Properties

Neither the sun nor death can be looked at with a steady eye.
—La Rochefoucauld

The political scientists Harold and Margaret Sprout, pioneers in the application of ecological principles to the domain of political science, noted that when complex connections exist between elements "any substantial change in one sector of the milieu is nearly certain to produce significant, often unsettling, sometimes utterly disruptive consequences in other sectors."[42] As such, tracing processes though case studies permits a holistic examination of the system wherein "the properties of the whole . . . can only be discovered by studying the whole."[43] The political scientist Robert Jervis concurs, arguing that systems are typically highly complex and contingent.[44] Jervis goes on to define the properties of a system:

We are dealing with a system when (a) the set of units or elements is interconnected so that changes in some elements or their relations produce changes in other parts of the system, and (b) the entire system exhibits properties and behaviors that are different from those of the parts. . . . The result is that systems often display nonlinear relationships, outcomes cannot be understood by adding together the units of their relations, and many of the results of actions are unintended. Complexities can appear even in what would appear to be simple and deterministic situations.[45]

Thus, natural systems exhibit profound complexity. Small changes that are gradually introduced over time may induce temporally distal nonlinearities, whereupon the system suddenly shifts to a new equilibrium.[46] Thus, human attempts to tame nature typically result in unforeseen negative outcomes. One notable example of such an outcome was the use of DDT to wipe out mosquitoes in order to diminish the transmission of such arthropod-borne diseases (e.g., malaria). Regrettably, the use of DDT resulted in widespread destruction of avian populations and generated evolutionary pressures that eventually created resistant populations of the vector.

The chains of connections among disparate elements (or variables) within a system may be exceedingly complex, often involving feedback loops and contingencies. The relationship among a pathogen, a vector, and a host is complex, and the debilitation or destruction of the human host will then generate externalities throughout a society that reverberate across various domains (e.g., demographic, psychological, economic, political). Indeed, outcomes in one domain may affect outcomes in other domains, creating feedback loops that perpetuate constant evolution of the system.[47] In addition, many bio-political systems may exhibit lag effects, wherein outcomes are delayed, are indirect, and intensify over the longer term.[48]

Furthermore, when examining the effects of disease on political structures, we may find that iterated indirect effects trump direct effects in their influence on systemic outcomes. Preliminary evidence suggests that the indirect effects of health on state capacity are attenuated and are likely to increase over the longer term.[49]

Aristotle acknowledged principles of non-linearity and randomness when he commented that "things do, in a way, occur by chance."[50] Variables within complex systems often interact to generate outcomes not predicted by linear models. Non-linear functions are often observed in natural systems, the obvious example being booms and subsequent crashes in the population of an animal species. Epidemiological curves also illustrate principles of non-linearity, wherein variables combine to generate exponential growth in the rates of infection, then plateau, and then crash as acquired immunity in the infected host population reaches a self-sustaining critical point.[51]

In his description of the SARS epidemic that struck Toronto in 2003, Justice Archie Campbell, Chief Commissioner of Canada's SARS Commission, described the contagion as a "perfect storm" of diverse factors.[52] This analogy is appropriate: epidemics often exhibit "emergent properties," in that the manifestation of contagion possesses characteristics that are greater and perhaps quite different than its constituent parts and that might be quite unexpected. As the sociologist Emile Durkheim commented, "whenever certain elements combine and thereby produce, by the fact of their new combination, new phenomena, it is plain that these new phenomena reside not in the original elements but in the totality formed by their union [or interaction]."[53] Thus, complex systems may exhibit properties that are attributable not to their discrete components, but rather to the macro-level interaction of those components, and thus (under conditions of strong emergence) the whole may be both greater than and different from the sum of its parts.[54]

Emerging pathogens, and their manifestations in epidemic or pandemic form, often exhibit "emergent properties" resulting from the interaction of variables in complex and interdependent global systems. The collectivity may not only be a function of the combination of direct effects of the discrete variables within a system; it may also be a function of unanticipated side effects of these variables. For example, population growth and increasing population density generates unanticipated side effects that permit the zoonotic transmission of disease into, and expansion throughout, the human ecology. The exceptionally dense and large aggregate populations of "mega-cities" can act as population pools that support the endogenous (and continuous) transmission of certain pathogens. The classic example of this is measles, which can maintain steady transmission rates only in cities with populations of at least 250,000.[55] Therefore, the rise of huge and concentrated new urban population centers, coupled with environmental degradation and rapid migration, may permit the endogenization of new pathogenic zoonoses (e.g., SARS) within the human ecology.

The concept of chaos is also applicable to evolutionary changes in the genetic structures of pathogenic agents. As the virologist Joshua Lederberg pointed out, the genetic structures of pathogens are highly mutable, and changes in traits of transmissibility and lethality are often governed by chance mutation.[56] The classic example is the influenza virus, whose genetic structure is constantly shifting and changing. The evolutionary trajectory of influenza is decidedly non-linear in nature and, consequently, highly unpredictable. As was demonstrated by the H5N1 variant of the virus, it could rapidly evolve into a lethal pandemic (along the lines of the 1918 "Spanish Flu") or it could simply mutate into a relatively benign and non-pathogenic variant (as happened with Swine Flu in 1976).

On the Utility of Punctuated-Equilibrium Theory

Jumps rather than smooth progressions often characterize operations of systems [and] when variables interact in a non-linear manner changes may not be gradual. Instead for a prolonged period there may be no apparent deterioration, followed by a sudden collapse or transformation.

—Robert Jervis[57]

For some time the dominant paradigms within political science have held that human societies (and their institutions of governance) exhibit linear trajectories of progression and/or decline, a process of functional, incremental change, and just "muddling through."[58] However, given that evolutionary change occurs in the natural world according to punctuated, and non-linear models, it seems reasonable to examine the hypothesis that punctuated-equilibrium (PE) models might interact with Schumpeterian theory to explain how non-linear disruptions may foster ingenuity, socio-political adaptation, and rapid institutional change in human societies. Conversely, if disease-induced requirements for ingenuity exceed endogenous adaptive capacity, protracted and widespread institutional breakdown may subsequently occur.[59]

At the domestic (or state) level, preliminary empirical evidence confirms that PE models possess a certain degree of validity. Stephen Krasner, one of the first political scientists to cast doubt on the incrementalist (i.e. functionalist) position, wrote that "studies of political development point to differential rates of change in social and political structures over time."[60] The political economist Douglass North discussed such possibilities of institutional transformation,[61] and the political scientists Frank Baumgartner and Bryan Jones found empirical evidence that PE models explained both the rate and the magnitude of change within US domestic political institutions.[62] In further empirical studies, the political scientists Speth and Repetto, Romanelli and Tushman, and Breunig and Koski all found positive evidence to support the premise of rapid and discontinuous change in institutions of governance.[63] The events of September 11, 2001 provide a powerful example of non-linear change in the US domestic apparatus of governance—change that led to the rapid re-constitution of various and disparate operations into the monolithic Department of Homeland Security. Those events also marked a profound transition in the conceptualization of US national security: non-state actors now were recognized as major threats, and terrorism rose to the top of the security agenda. September 11 also prompted a significant shift in US foreign policy toward pre-emptive war, the neoconservative (ultimately Kantian) promotion of democracy through war, and US intervention in Iraq and Afghanistan. Thus, one exceptional and unanticipated event triggered a flurry of rapid and wide-ranging changes in the United States' structure of governance, and in its patterns of behavior in the international system.

Historically, the study of international relations (a subset of political science) has been marked by the persistence of linear and incremental orthodoxy, yet challenges to this dogma have arisen in recent years. The political scientist Mark Blyth argues that the emergence of novel ideas propelled rapid and non-linear institutional and economic change in Europe and North America throughout the twentieth century.[64] James Rosenau notes that the "the emergent world is marked by a high degree of disorder and turbulence," and that "the dynamics of turbulence penetrate to the very core of the human experience."[65] Further, Rosenau argues that political analysts have been perennial "prisoners of their theories," and that "the tendency to highlight continuities stems from excessive caution and a lack of clarity as to the nature of anomalies."[66] Additionally, the political scientists Paul Diehl and Gary Goertz explicitly employ PE models to explain the onset and termination of international conflict over the centuries.[67]

The exogenous shock of war can, depending on the adaptive capacity of the polities involved, generate enormous incentives for ingenuity, restructuring, and adaptation. Indeed, the historical record suggests that war often generates profound and rapid transformations both within the affected sovereign states and in international relations. Conversely, if the power of the shock exceeds the adaptive capacity of the affected polity, it will destabilize that system, and in extreme cases it will induce the collapse of that polity. Historical examples of the exogenous shock of war (both inter-state and intra-state) as a driver of state collapse and/or systemic transformation abound. In the twentieth century alone, one need only look at the two world wars to comprehend this notion of punctuated-equilibrium dynamics as the drivers of change at both the domestic and systems levels. World War I is particularly interesting, as it resulted in the political transmogrification of Imperial Germany into a nascent (and brittle) democracy, induced the dissolution of Austria-Hungary and the Ottoman Empire, and laid the foundation for World War II. That war, arguably more destructive than its predecessor, resulted in the division of Germany, the effective end of Britain's and France's imperial ambitions, and the shift of global power away from Europe to Washington and Moscow. World War II also generated social ingenuity: the global economic system was reformed (under the Bretton Woods agreement), and the United Nations was created to preclude such a destructive conflict in the future.

Given that the exogenous shock of war can function to generate either adaptation or destruction at the state and systems levels, it behooves us to explore the possibility that epidemics of disease may have historically functioned in a similar fashion. The bubonic plague that stalked European populations from 1348 until the mid 1700s, destroying an estimated 25–33 percent of Europe's population, may qualify as a series of exogenous shocks.[68] Pathogenic waves were generated by exogenous agents (bacilli) that traveled via vectors (rats and fleas) into the human ecology, where they generated extreme morbidity and mortality. As I will argue in chapter 2, the pathogenic waves generated by the Black Death generated enormous social, economic, and political instability, led to significant transformations within European polities, and directly contributed to the demise of the feudal system. In the Americas, the catastrophic devastation wrought by smallpox on immunologically naive Amerindian populations overwhelmed the adaptive capacity of the Aztec and Incan empires and directly facilitated their subsequent conquest by European forces.

The utility of the PE model lies in its capacity to explain rapid and non-linear shifts within political systems, be they global (such as the rapid collapse of the bipolar structure of the Cold War era) or domestic systems of governance. Such models account for the rapid destabilization or transformation of states and/or systems, and cast doubt on incrementalist orthodoxy. In the domain of health and governance, PE models suggest that incremental increases in infection rates over time may produce negative and concatenating effects across domains within a system, gradually increasing the stresses on that polity. Eventually incidence or prevalence of a pathogen may cross a threshold, after which rapid and non-linear change is observed in the affected system. If a polity possesses sufficient endogenous adaptive capacity and ingenuity,[69] then successful adaptation will occur, and rapid and positive institutional change is likely. On the other hand, if a polity's resilience and capacity are insufficient, the pathogen may overwhelm existing structures (socioeconomic and political) and precipitate significant instability throughout the system, followed by a new equilibrium that may be very different from the one that preceded it.

On Cognition, Affect, and Construction

Positivist thought holds that there is an empirical reality to epidemic disease, and that pathogens and disease can be measured, manipulated, and observed. However, it also seems reasonable to argue that human beings may perceive this "objective" reality in very "subjective" ways, which may vary across individuals and across societies. The medical historian Sheldon Watts concurs, noting that "humans are biological entities (we are an animal type known among ourselves as *Homo sapiens sapiens*), while at the same time we are bearers of culture."[70] There is a common ground between the extremes of constructivism and positivism on this subject, and the starting point is to admit that the overwhelming balance of empirical evidence demonstrates that pathogens exist as distinct and independent organisms that generate destructive effects on their hosts. Pathogens exist as independent (exogenous) empirical entities, and can thrive both within and outside of human societies. And many such agents function as zoonoses which have crossed over into the human ecology from their natural animal reservoirs.

Yet the concepts of disease and "illness" of the host may be interpreted (and indeed fashioned in certain respects) by society. The perception of disease and the processes of cognition will condition a society's response to infectious disease both at the individual level and at the collective level. The social sciences inform the debate by illuminating the causal effects of economic and societal inequities on the pathogen-host relationship, as such inequities (e.g., poverty-induced malnutrition) may in fact weaken the host and make the host more vulnerable to colonization by microbial agents. Thus, epidemics may also be regarded as "constructs" wherein the original damage of the pathogen is exacerbated through human perceptions (and misperceptions), the intrusion of affect (fear in particular), stigmatization of the infected, and overreaction by the state (which has often resulted in draconian measures that have exacerbated or produced societal destabilizations). Watts notes this lingering tension between epistemic communities, and argues that "disease" is a reality (synonymous with disease agent/pathogen) whereas "illness" is—at least in part—a perception. " 'Illness' (as perceived by 'self') can be caused by *individual* misfortune and circumstances."[71] The historian Paul Slack validates this synthesis of views, arguing that "different microorganisms affect their human hosts and human societies in different ways. Yet epidemics are also themselves intellectual 'constructs' which, once formulated, have a history, vitality, and resilience of their own."[72] Thus, acceptance of the empirical basis of epidemics, and of its subsequent interpretation, allows us to bridge the epistemic divide between the social sciences and the natural sciences, and to advance the scholarly debate.

On Fear as Mechanism

Disease-induced morbidity and mortality produces quantifiable negative effects on human capital and reduces the productivity of workers, but economic damage and violence between societal factions may also be induced by the visceral fear of contagion. Fear and anxiety generated by infectious disease may generate responses ranging from Pareto-suboptimal decision making to denial to social dissolution to vicious persecution of minorities or of other polities. Destabilization resulting from fear and anxiety may even lead to the oppression of the people by a governmental apparatus of coercion in order to maintain the ideology of order and the "interests" of the state.

Humans, therefore, tend to exhibit bounded rationality, wherein the individual seeks to act rationally under various cognitive and affective constraints. Deudney concurs, noting the profound role of fear as a driver of international politics, particularly in matters of security:

> ... human rationality is a relatively frail faculty of the human psyche and easily overpowered by the various emotions, most notably fear and anger. Fear is the emotion most intimately linked to security, and how fear is managed—expressed, repressed, directed, or cultivated—is among the most elemental issues of security politics. The dynamics of fear are central to many of the most influential analyses of political security. . . . When human beings are gripped by the emotion of fear their capacity for instrumental rationality is often impaired. As Thucydides so vividly shows, fear can lead individuals and groups to take actions that are panicked and ill-conceived.[73]

The history of contagion suggests that instrumental rationality is often at a premium during episodes of contagion, wherein the visitation of an epidemic generated enormous levels of affect (emotions of fear and anxiety) that heralded social polarization and generated inter-ethnic and inter-class strife. While the bodies of the deceased accumulated, further destabilization arose through misperception and the creation of images[74] of the "ill" and of the carriers of illness (vectors). Such emotional responses require us to re-think previously dominant models of cold cognition, and to postulate that hot-cognitive models (which include the role of affect) are required to explain societal, political, and indeed economic responses to epidemic disease.[75]

Cognitive factors may also inhibit the human capacity to accurately assess risks associated with the emergence of novel pathogens. As the legal scholar Richard Posner notes, individuals tend to overweight risks associated with phenomena that are considered "dreadful" and "unknown," such as emergent diseases.[76] In addition, Posner argues that humans exhibit "imagination cost," which is a "difficulty in thinking about things that lie outside one's experience."[77] The legal scholar Cass Sunstein argues that the inaccurate assessment of such risk often stems from "probability neglect," which is the persistent inability of most humans to respond in rational fashion to dire risks with very low probabilities.[78] It may be completely rational for human beings to avoid a pathogenic agent that may cause their untimely death or debilitation. Such behavior might be described as prudent risk aversion. The problem lies within the individual's capacity to correctly evaluate a novel pathogen's potential to generate death and debilitation.

The epistemic community of experts on public health is very small. The average citizen has a very limited capacity to make Pareto-optimal rational decisions about risks associated with a pathogen's transmissibility and lethality, or about the availability of prophylactics or countermeasures. In the event of the emergence of novel pathogens, even public health experts will lack such information for a protracted period, and so extreme uncertainty results in profound levels of fear and anxiety, which typically results in significant displays of affect-induced irrational behavior. Fear of contagion can also generate or exacerbate in-group/out-group identity formation, resulting in the scapegoating of "others" and often in the intensification of xenophobia and racism. Thus, fear is notably enhanced by the uncertainty associated with the pathogenic agent in question. The SARS epidemic of 2002–03 was such an epidemic of fear, generated by the great levels of uncertainty about the etiology of the pathogen, its vectors of transmission, its possible communicability and virulence, and the efficacy (or lack thereof) of possible prophylactics and treatments.

2

Epidemic Disease, History, and the State

The history of life, like that of humanity, flows through a channel confined by the edicts of nature. . . .
—William Rosen

Times of plague are always those in which the bestial and diabolical side of human nature gains the upper hand.
—Barthold Georg Neibuhr

"Salus populi suprema lex esto," Cicero advised his patrons among the ruling elites of Rome. Translated, this approximates "The welfare of the people shall be the supreme law."[1] Thus, the health and well-being of the population forms the very foundation of prosperity, of political stability, and indeed of the power of disparate societies relative to one another. If the welfare of the people is paramount, then those pathogenic forces that would undermine human well-being should be regarded as distinct threats to the cohesion, material interests and power of the state.

Over the span of recorded human history, the proliferation of infectious disease has acted as a stressor, generating significant and profound destabilization of societies and polities. Historians and anthropologists have increasingly recognized disease as a variable that has affected historical outcomes, in some cases considerably.[2] Only belatedly have such connections between the natural and social sciences been revisited by political theorists.[3] However, republican and Classical Realist theories of international politics have contained the seeds of such knowledge since the earliest writings in that disciplinary genre.

This chapter reviews the role of disease in the destabilization of societies, economies, and sovereign states from ancient Athens to the modern era (1914 AD). Pathogens are an ancient phenomenon. (Poliomyelitis virus was found in a Neolithic skeleton from Cissbury, Sussex, England.) Further, the bacterium that induces tuberculosis first appears in textual references in the Egyptian Ebers medical papyrus and in the Rig Veda, both dated to circa 1500 BC. Paleopathological evidence culled from human remains suggests that the pathogen existed in Italy during the fourth millennium BC. The pestilence, chronicled in the works of Hippocrates and Avicenna, flourished on a continental scale during the reign of Edward the Confessor in England (1003–1066 AD).[4] *Treponema* bacteria, some of which induce syphilis, have been discovered in human remains in Siberia and dated to 1000 BC, and syphilis is evident in the skeletal remains of the Americas predating the arrival of Columbus. Material evidence of syphilis does not appear in Europe until 1500 AD, which supports the hypothesis that it was transported to the Old World via the Columbian Exchange.[5]

Each pathogen, with its unique niche in the human ecology, generates a constellation of diverse effects on affected countries. Thus, this chapter analyzes the effect of individual pathogens on state-society interactions over the historical record. The historical record compiled here indicates that contagion may foment significant socio-political instability, and I conclude from the balance of evidence that infectious diseases have historically represented a significant threat to the cohesion, the interests, the power, and thus the security of the state.

The pursuit of interdisciplinary (or consilient[6]) thought represents the epistemological basis of this volume, and therefore I eschew the "silo mentality" or fragmentation of knowledge arising from acute disciplinary specialization in the modern era. The political historian John Gaddis argues vociferously against this "Balkanization" of the disciplines: ". . . we have been known, from time to time, to construct the intellectual equivalent of fortified trenches from which we fire artillery back and forth, dodging shrapnel even as we sink ever more deeply into mutual incomprehension."[7] Further, Gaddis argues that history and political science share a common intellectual ancestry, and he bemoans the "narcissism of minor differences" that, over the past century, has driven the disciplines apart. The political scientist Harvey Mansfield echoes this view: "My profession needs to open its eyes and admit to its curriculum the help of literature and history. It should be unafraid to risk considering what is ignored by science and may lack the approval of science."[8]

The effects of epidemic disease on societies, economies, and polities throughout history may inform our understanding of the effects of contagion on modern peoples. Thus, historical precedents form the basis of our postulates regarding the effects of contagion on modern state-society interactions. Therefore, it is reasonable to assume that the significant work of historians, over the centuries, might provide political scientists with a wealth of qualitative observations from which to derive certain hypotheses regarding the effects of infectious disease on structures of governance. Such historical luminaries as Procopius,[9] Galen,[10] and Hippocrates[11] recorded their direct observations regarding the destructive influence of contagion on prosperity and socio-political stability. One of the earliest records of the destabilizing effect of contagion comes from the Athenian general and historian Thucydides, who noted the highly destructive effects of the "plague" on Athenian social stability and power in his account of the Peloponnesian War.[12] Subsequently, another father of republican thought (and subsequently Realist theory)— the Italian provocateur Niccolo Machiavelli—chronicled the socio-political and economic disruptions he witnessed during the plague's visitation to Florence in 1527. "Our pitiful Florence," Machiavelli wrote acridly,

now looks like nothing but a town which has been stormed by the infidels and then forsaken. One part of the inhabitants . . . have retired to the distant country houses; one part is dead, and yet another part is dying. Thus the present is torment, the future menace, so we contend with death and only live in fear and trembling. The clean fine streets which formerly teemed with rich and noble citizens are now stinking and dirty. . . . Shops and inns are closed, at the factories work has ceased, the law courts are empty, the laws are trampled on. The squares, the market places of which the citizens used frequently to assemble, have now been converted into graves and into the resort of a wicked rabble.[13]

Modern conceptualizations that link the emergence and proliferation of pathogens to the destabilization of a polity can be found in the works of the historians William McNeill, Alfred Crosby, Hans Zinsser, Sheldon Watts, and Michael Oldstone. It is curious that the pernicious effects of epidemics on states and societies should be well established in the domain of history and yet be paid little attention in the domain of political science. This lacuna in the latter discipline may be attributable to the nascent nature of political science, emerging as it did during the twentieth century, when outbreaks of contagion were increasingly constrained by the development of antibiotics.

The medical historian Hans Zinsser argues that negative externalities associated with contagion were not measured merely through mortality, but that they instilled profound disorganization into the affected polity in question.[14] The visitation of contagion on a population generated significant levels of trepidation, often inspiring the mass flight of individuals from affected regions. Zinsser notes the pernicious affects of such fear on the affected polity: "Panic bred social and moral disorganization; farms were abandoned, and there was shortage of food; famine led to displacement of populations, to revolution, to civil war, and, in some instances, to fanatical religious movements which contributed to profound spiritual and political transformations."[15] The historical evidence provided below reinforces many of the theoretical postulates I have provided in the preceding chapter, and it provides us a referent point to assess the degree to which the relations between contagion and the state-societies dynamic have persisted into the modern era.

Let us now briefly examine a selection of specific pathogens and their deleterious economic, social, and political effects on polities, from ancient times to the early twentieth century.

Typhus

The word "typhus" is derived from the Greek *typhos*, which means "hazy" or "smoky" (referring to the victim's mental state). The illness, caused by bacteria of the *Rickettsia* class, was an ancient bane of both cities and armies, exploding throughout dense human populations courtesy of its ubiquitous vectors: the louse, the flea, and the rat.[16] As I have already noted, Thucydides, in his classic account of the travails experienced during the Peloponnesian War, chronicled the debilitating effect of the "plague of Athens" (i.e., typhus) on Athenian society.[17] The contagion emerged out of Ethiopia and struck Athens in 430 BC, returning in 429 BC to take the life of the Athenian leader Pericles and thus to erode the political cohesion of the polity. Medical historians, notably David Durack, have concluded that clinical manifestations of typhus are most representative of the contagion that ravaged Athens.[18] However, recent forensic epidemiological investigations by the Greek dental physician Manolis Papagrigorakis[19] suggest that the contagion that struck Athens may have been typhoid fever rather than typhus.[20] The debate continues, but it is quite possible that both pathogens existed in the same population at the same time.

While the exact nature of the pathogen is debated, historians have fashioned a consensus that the "plague" generated profoundly destabilizing effects on Athenian social cohesion, governance, and power during the protracted conflict with Sparta and her allies. As Thucydides noted, the epidemic that coursed through Athens generated a significant disruption of social norms, undermined the observation of existing laws, and ultimately had a markedly deleterious effect on governance:

The bodies of the dying were heaped one on top of the other, and half-dead creatures could be seen staggering about in the streets or flocking around the fountains in their desire for water. For the catastrophe was so overwhelming that men, not knowing what would next happen to them, became indifferent to every rule of religion or law. Athens owed to the plague the beginnings of a state of unprecedented lawlessness. Seeing how quick and abrupt were the changes of fortune . . . people now began openly to venture on acts of self-indulgence which before then they used to keep in the dark. As for what is called honor, no one showed himself willing to abide by its laws, so doubtful was it whether one would survive to enjoy the name for it. No fear of god nor law of man had a restraining influence. As for the gods, it seemed to be the same thing whether one worshipped them or not, when one saw the good and the bad dying indiscriminately. As for offences against human law, no one expected to live long enough to be brought to trial and punished.[21]

According to estimates by the historian James Longrigg, the waves of contagion killed approximately one-third of the population of Athens, and during the second outbreak of contagion 4,400 hoplites (heavily armed foot soldiers) died, out of a total of 13,000, while 300 of 1,000 cavalry were killed from the pathogen in question.[22] The historian A. W. Gomme, who analyzed Athenian accounts of the contagion, determined that the epidemic resulted in the destruction of roughly one-third of Athens' land-based military forces.[23] William McNeill and Hans Zinsser argue that the contagion fundamentally undermined Athenian power, and speculate that it may have altered the historical outcome of the conflict.[24] Longrigg concurs:

Thucydides has realized the important role played by the impact of the plague in Athens' ultimate defeat. Not only did the plague have a serious adverse effect upon Athenian military man-power; but it also, Thucydides believes, adversely affected, both directly and indirectly, Athenian leadership and policy during the war. Pericles, it seems, died of the plague and, it appears Alcibiades was later impeached under legislation introduced during and as a result of the plague. Thucydides has recognized . . . the importance of medical factors in the history of warfare.[25]

The consequent demographic collapse of the armed forces, the crippling of Athenian political elites, and the debilitation and demoralization of a significant proportion of the survivors certainly diminished Athens' capacity to project power (martial and ideological) against Sparta and her allies.[26]

Plague (*Yersinia pestis*)

McNeill argues that the destruction of the Byzantine Roman empire in the sixth century AD was wrought by the "plague of Justinian," arguably the first visitation of *Yersinia pestis* to Europe.[27] The Plague acted as a stressor or a solvent on the machinery of empire, resulting in the attenuated erosion of societal and state cohesion, prosperity, and power during the sixth century AD. This emergent pathogen was one of the first negative consequences of the early phases of "globalization," as trade and migration along the Silk Road saw the dissemination of *Yersinia pestis* from its natural reservoirs in Central Asia to Europe and East Asia.[28] Consequently, the contagion resulted in massive mortality among immunologically naive populations throughout the Mediterranean region.[29] The demographer Josiah Russell has argued that all the available data indicate that before the arrival of the contagion the populations of the Byzantine Roman Empire and the Persian Empire were robust and enjoying a rapid rate of increase.[30] According to the historian William Rosen, this particular manifestation of contagion claimed the lives of circa 25 million people in and around the Mediterranean basin. Rosen concurs with Russell that it "depopulated entire cities; and depressed birth rates for generations precisely at the time that Justinian's armies had returned the entire Western Mediterranean to imperial control."[31]

Procopius wrote that he witnessed the Plague-induced destruction of 10,000 persons per day at Constantinople, where the illness raged for approximately four months.[32] He also noted the profound psychological effects of the illness on norms of behavior and social cohesion. "And after the plague had ceased, there was so much depravity and general licentiousness, that it seemed as though the disease had left only the most wicked."[33] Gibbon's account of the disruptive effects of the contagion accords with Procopius' observations:

I only find that, during three months, five and at length ten thousand persons died each day at Constantinople; and many cities of the east were left vacant, and that in several districts of Italy the harvest and the vintage withered on the ground. The triple scourges of war, pestilence and famine afflicted the subjects of Justinian; and his reign is disgraced by a visible decrease of the human species which has never been regained in some of the fairest countries of the globe.[34]

According to Russell, the initial wave of plague (541–544 AD) reduced the population around the Mediterranean (European and otherwise) by 20–25 percent over a three-year period.[35] The contagion also served to induce the collapse of agricultural productivity, as pronounced demographic contraction induced severe labor shortages. John of Ephesus noted that "in every field from Syria to Thrace the harvest lacked a harvester."[36]

This scenario was replicated in non-European lands. The demographers Ronald Findlay and Mats Lundahl write: "It is a fact (although some historians still refuse to recognize it) that all around the Mediterranean, the cities, as they had existed in antiquity, contracted and then practically disappeared."[37] The historian Michael Dols argues that epidemic disease often destabilized existing socio-political and economic equilibria, but that it also contained catalytic potential for the transformation of state-society relations following periods of exceptional turbulence:

... the pandemic and its recurrent epidemics were the solvents of classical Mediterranean civilization and were largely responsible for the formation of new political, social, and economic patterns ... political power gradually shifted to the peoples of northern Europe, who were relatively unaffected by the epidemics, and, conversely, plague greatly weakened the Byzantine empire. Justinian's plans for re-establishing the Roman Empire were wrecked, and the diminished Byzantine armies were unable to defend the extensive frontiers. Hence, there was the successful resurgence of barbarian invasions. . . .[38]

McNeill, Zinsser, and Rosen support this conceptualization of the Fall of Byzantium, concurring that the stresses generated on both state and society overwhelmed the Empire's adaptive capacity, its ability to defend itself, and its ability to project martial power against its rivals, and led to the polity's gradual dissolution.[39]

The negative effects of contagion on governance and power projection were consequential, and they were hardly confined to the Mediterranean region. Indeed, it appears that East Asian societies suffered similarly destabilizing effects when the contagion reached them centuries later. McNeill argues that, in the wake of a military revolt in 755 AD, the dissolution of central political authority in China was temporally synchronous with the waves of bubonic plague that visited the region.[40]

The Black Death: 1348

Beginning in 1348, *Yersinia pestis* (in its various bubonic, pneumonic, and septicemic manifestations) again visited Europe and the Middle East. The waves of contagion that became known as the Black Death swept across the entire region and again diminished the now immunologically naive population.[41] The spread of disease was accompanied by profound fear and anxiety, giving rise to a host of odd (and often destructive) responses by affected populations. The geographer Harold Foster has ranked the appearance of the Black Death in Europe as the second-worst catastrophe in human history, superseded only by World War II in absolute destructive capacity.[42] Estimates of contagion-induced mortality in affected populations range from 5 percent to 50 percent.[43] However, the consensus figure is that 30–45 percent of Europe's population was destroyed by the contagion.[44]

The epidemic generated moral, socio-political, and economic disintegration. It also generated mass flight from urban centers to safer rural areas, leading to the depopulation of urban areas. Paul Slack argues that contagion-induced flight from affected areas constitutes a fundamental historical axiom of societal responses but that it carried negative consequences for societal cohesion, and for effective governance, "since it took people away from charitable, neighborly, or political duties."[45] Manifestations of the contagion in Egypt resulted in a different dynamic as the rapid depopulation of rural (agrarian) areas led to famine, which consequently intensified the depopulation of the cities.[46] Sheldon Watts further describes the effects of plague on other regions of Egypt: ". . . at Luxor, of the 24,000 feddans of arable land under crops before 1347, only 1,000 were still being cultivated in 1389."[47] Thus was Cairo rapidly emptied and impoverished by the Black Death.[48]

Emulating the earlier destabilization of Byzantium, Dols argues, the Black Death effectively eroded the cohesion, prosperity, and power of the Mamluk Empire, leading to its dissolution. Dols argues that declines in agricultural productivity diminished the flows of revenues to the Mamluk elites, and consequently to the central government's investment in irrigation and other rural infrastructure, leading to the disintegration of the empire.[49] The historian David Ayalon argued that the aggregate effect of waves of plague in Egypt was severe deterioration of the Mamluk armies, and a corresponding decline of Mamluk military power throughout the late fourteenth century, which led directly to the Ottoman conquest of Egypt.[50]

Thus, the Black Death exhibited the capacity to generate pernicious effects on regional economies, as the destruction of the population eroded the existing base of human capital, and thereby diminished economic productivity.[51] Moreover, the Black Death disrupted wage and price patterns, generating economic contraction, which in turn exacerbated conflict between classes in prosperous regions such as Flanders and northern Italy.[52] In addition, manifestations of plague disrupted trade flows, and ultimately shifted regional balances of economic power from the affected city-states to unaffected regions:

> While Venice was closed down and its plague-dead leadership was being replenished from youthful entries in its Golden Book. . . . Dutch and English entrepreneurs moved into its traditional marketing territories around the Adriatic and Eastern Mediterranean. Once in possession they stayed. Shorn of its major markets and burdened with leaders suffering from sclerosis (young in body but old in mind), Venice soon found itself only a regional power with no economic clout. From this it was but a short step to becoming a museum city.[53]

The negative effects of the Black Death on social cohesion and on governance were also pronounced. The medical historian Johannes Nohl argues that conditions of privation, as directly fostered by the contagion, resulted in a terrible degradation of morality and social stability during this era of European history.[54] During the affliction of Paris 1468, the French surgeon Ambroise Pare observed that the state's capacity for effective governance was dramatically eroded by the contagion: "The worst of all is that the rich, the higher town officials and all persons vested with official authority, flee among the first at the outbreak of the plague. . . . General anarchy and confusion then set in and that is the worst evil by which the commonwealth can be assailed."[55] As in the case of cholera, the perceived legitimacy of government institutions was compromised by the contagion, as relations between classes deteriorated and the peasantry actively resisted the proclamations of government officials.[56]

Within the broader European context, the plague generated significant inter-ethnic hostility, exacerbating tensions between European gentiles and the resident Jewish and Roma populations.[57] Plague was also responsible for exacerbating pre-existing inter-ethnic tensions, manifesting in the scapegoating and often torture of minorities. Exceptional violence was directed by panicked Christian populations against Jewish minorities throughout Europe during this period. Anti-Jewish pogroms were carried out throughout Europe, and with a particular intensity in France and Germany, largely as a result of the dissemination of conspiracy theories that the Jews were poisoning the wells of Christian communities. The fact that Jews too died of plague did nothing to dissuade many from adopting such outlandish theories and engaging in violence against the now vilified minority.[58] The Black Death, Slack argues, "provoked extreme religious reactions, including a revival of eschatological prophecies. . . . The Christian notions of original sin and divine chastisement therefore predisposed men to action: to search out the targets of epidemics, often to find scapegoats, but also to identify the physical as well as the moral sources of disease—unruly public assemblies, vagrants and beggars, disorderly slums."[59]

One of the first cases of plague inspired the pogroms that occurred in May 1348 in Provence.[60] Pogroms then occurred across Europe for decades, and draconian legislation, such as that enacted in Strasbourg in 1348, ensured the continued persecution of Jews.[61] However, this pales in comparison to the atrocities committed at Basle. "The diabolical scheme," Nohl writes, "was then conceived of imprisoning all Jews in a wooden shed on an island in the Rhine, outside the town, and then setting the shed on fire. . . . These atrocities were perpetrated exclusively on the tempestuous urging of the populace. . . ."[62]

The xenophobia and targeting of minorities during times of plague was not relegated solely to the targeting of Jews and Roma. In Spain in 1630 the French were designated as the "poisoners," and they were subsequently targeted as convenient scapegoats. "In consequence of this," Nohl writes, "all Frenchmen . . . became . . . unpopular. . . . Ultimately a royal edict was issued that all Frenchmen in Spain had to be registered."[63] The plague also gave rise to unusual behaviors and disruptive groups, such as the Flagellants, who beat themselves to stave off the wrath of the divine for their prior sins and who sought to undermine the authority of the Roman Catholic Church.[64]

During Britain's occupation and colonization of the Indian subcontinent, the recrudescence of *Yersinia pestis* also exacerbated ethnic tensions between the British overseers and their indigenous subjects and induced societal destabilization[65]:

People found themselves pitted against each other in the panic far more than they were gathered into large social solidarities. Social tension, competition and antagonisms were heightened not only between but also within classes. The fragile façade of social order was cracked open and whole towns and villages appeared to be on the edge of chaos. In virtually every town, the outbreak of plague paralyzed trade and put its inhabitants to flight. At anarchy's edge, the panic created fresh opportunities for profit and power for those with the temerity and ruthlessness to seize them. The evacuation of towns and villages . . . was accompanied by an increased incidence, and fear, of crime.[66]

The cumulative impact of waves of plague generated profound changes in relations between the state and society in Europe. The proliferation of contagion certainly generated significant lawlessness, inter-ethnic violence, and changes in accepted norms of behavior. In addition, it often undermined the capacity of governmental institutions to provide services to the people, damaging the state's legitimacy. Such sclerotic effects of the plague resulted in declining economic productivity, diminishing tax revenues available to the state, which in turn resulted in further weakening of armies and police forces. The force of the plague even undermined the cohesion of institutions of higher learning, such as Oxford University.[67] The societal disarray that accompanied visitations of *la peste* often generated correspondingly draconian reactions by the state against the people in order to maintain order, eventually causing erosion of governmental legitimacy and a shift in power toward the state and away from the society it claimed to protect.

Perhaps the most notable outcome of the waves of plague was the creation of an ideology of coercion that concentrated power in the hands of the state in order to control the people. In this manner, epidemic diseases have often generated a shift in power away from the people and toward the apparatus of coercion, often resulting in oppression of the people in order to guarantee order. The quarantinist ideology, also known as contagionism, often mandated harsh laws that tended to inflame tensions between state and society. The period of the Black Death gave rise to the first structures of public health governance, notably in the Italian city-states of Venice and Florence and subsequently in Milan (where public health commissions were constituted in 1348). Public health commissions gradually evolved into permanent institutions that monitored public health,[68] setting a precedent that would be emulated by other city-states over the centuries. The practice of the quarantine of maritime vessels originated in Venice on March 20, 1348, continuing a tradition (dating from 1000 AD) of guarding the health of the people in order to protect the interests of both society and state.[69] The term "quarantine" (which refers to a 40-day period of sequestration) is derived from the Italian *quarantenaria*. Measures of quarantine to control the flows of infected goods and the isolation of the sick, developed by Bernabo Visconti, Duke of Milan, were first put into practice in Mantua and Raguso in 1374. The practice subsequently spread throughout Italy and then to the French port of Marseilles, which began to quarantine goods and travelers in 1383.[70]

During the late 1300s, the city of Firenze (Florence) followed the contagionist model of pathogenic containment, now well established in the north of Italy. According to the dictates of the ascendant Florentine Board of Health, during an outbreak of plague it became standard practice for military forces to ensure order in the towns of the region, and those who sought to slip through the military *cordon sanitaire* were routinely executed. Furthermore, the health administrators in Firenze made it necessary for people to carry "health passports" (declaring they were free of plague) to travel from one town to another.[71] Such coercion in the name of order was popular among the city-states of Italy, and from 1578 on this new authoritarianism was adopted in England. As Watts notes, "in England in 1604 anyone thought to have the plague who was found out on the streets could legally be hanged."[72]

In seventeenth-century Tuscany such draconian public health laws entailed sending individuals off to "pesthouses," locking entire families up in their homes, burning infected goods, shutting down markets, and suspending trade, which in turn fostered unemployment.[73] In 1679, Spain, adopting the Florentine model, imposed harsh controls on population movements, employing martial force to control migration between infected and disease-free zones.[74] The Habsburg regime instituted draconian restrictions on population movements throughout Central Europe in 1739 when it created "plague-control zones" in which military forces were under orders to fire on unauthorized travelers. Such *cordons sanitaires* covered the majority of Slavonia and Croatia, Transylvania, and various regions to the south of the Danube.[75]

The successive waves of bubonic plague that swept Europe from the fourteenth century through the early seventeenth century acted as a profound stressor on the feudal system. The rich and the poor, the pious and the heretic, all died in similar fashion, and so a fundamental axiom of epidemic disease became visible: the de-legitimization of existing hierarchies and structures of authority. In this case, the plague generated significant doubts about divine power, and therefore about the legitimacy of the Roman Catholic Church. Therefore, the successive waves of contagion and death gradually de-legitimized the pre-existing structures of religious authority throughout feudal societies in Europe.[76] This disease-induced mass destabilization and the de-legitimization of the Church contributed to the Protestant Reformation and thereby helped to fashion the tinderbox of pan-European conflagration known as the Thirty Years' War.[77]

Notwithstanding the minor outbreak of plague that occurred in Surat, India in 1994, the last significant outbreak of "plague" would seem to have occurred throughout India from 1896 to 1914. The historian Chandavarkar notes that the epidemic generated exceptional levels of affect (fear and panic), the social destabilization in turn resulting in the intervention of the state, which provoked "fierce resistance, riots, occasionally mob attacks on Europeans and even the assassination of British officials."[78] The epidemic, and the fear and social chaos it generated, compelled the British government to institute draconian measures and controls, including mass quarantine and the burning of personal property, and to construct a surveillance system replete with checkpoints and detention camps.[79] The British response was based on their perceptions that the emergence of plague in India constituted a direct threat to the material interests (i.e. prosperity), the power, and even the security of the Empire. Chandavarkar explains the "imperial consequences" of the plague as follows: "An international embargo on Indian shipping not only threatened to close an important market and source of raw materials for Britain but also disturb the intricate system for the multilateral settlement of its balance of payments, in which India played a large and vital part. If (the plague) spread through the subcontinent it might devastate India's social order and economic base, flatten the pivot of empire and undermine the foundation of Britain's influence between the Yellow and the Red Seas."[80]

Smallpox (*Variola major*)

The earliest empirical evidence of smallpox (the disease generated by the virus *Variola major*) dates from the preserved physical attributes of several Egyptian mummies. The most notable cadaver in this respect is that of Ramses V, who died in 1157 BC.[81] The disease would seem to have been subsequently transmitted to India circa 1150 BC, and thereafter to China in 1122 BC. The historian Jonathan Tucker suggests that smallpox played a significant role in the destruction of the army of Alexander the Great during his expedition to India, and that Marcus Aurelius succumbed to the contagion during the Antonine plague in 180 AD.[82]

The "Plague" of Antonius (165–180 AD), which appears to have been induced by *Variola*, had negative effects on the socio-economic stability and governance of Rome. The epidemic appears to have begun in the Roman army of Verus, which was conquering cities throughout Asia Minor in 165 AD. As the Roman forces returned to southern Europe, they distributed the contagion throughout the lands they traversed, eventually bringing it to Rome, whereupon Verus fell to the contagion in 169 AD. The historian Donald Hopkins argues that the illness claimed between 3.5 million and 7 million lives and "must have weakened the Empire."[83] Doubtless the contagion functioned as a significant stressor to erode the power of Rome. "There can be little room for doubt," Zinsser concludes, "that a calamity of this kind, lasting for over a decade, during a political period rendered critical by internal strife and constant war against encircling hostile barbarians, must have had a profound effect on the maintenance of the Roman power. Military campaigns were stopped, cities depopulated, agriculture all but destroyed, and commerce paralyzed."[84]

Smallpox generated further political discord by disrupting lines of succession throughout the ranks of European nobility. For example, in northern Italy, the Duke of Mantua and his only son succumbed to smallpox in December 1612. Abruptly ending the male line of succession of the Gonzaga family, this led directly to the War of the Mantuan Succession between Austria and France.[85]

In 1700 AD the pox raged in Britain, killing Queen Anne's only son, destroying the English royal house of Stuart,[86] and generating a constitutional crisis that ended in the Act of Settlement, which explicitly prohibited Catholics from occupying the throne and thereby opened the door to the Hanovers. The pox also disrupted the Habsburg dynasty, killing Emperor Joseph I in April 1711 and depriving the family of the Spanish succession. "Because Joseph I died without a son," Hopkins notes, "he was succeeded by his only surviving brother Charles VI. . . . By accepting the Austrian inheritance, Charles was forced to abandon the Spanish throne to the Bourbon claimant Philip V. Austria's erstwhile allies . . . now changed sides to support Philip V. . . ."[87] Various crowned heads of Europe fell to the pox, including Queen Mary II of England in 1694, Joseph I of Germany, King Louis I of Spain in 1724, Tsar Peter II of Russia in 1730, Queen Ulrika Eleanor of Sweden in 1741, King Louis XV of France in 1774, and William II of Orange.[88]

As I have already noted, early forms of globalization (conquest and trade) served as highly efficient vectors for the global spread of contagion, including *Variola*. The dissemination of pathogens throughout the Americas by European forces generated significant morbidity and mortality among indigenous peoples, and the consequent demographic implosion effectively undermined pre-existing structures of authority throughout Amerindian societies. This, in turn, facilitated the rapid conquest of the Americas and the extension of European empire.

The first reports of the pox in the Americas come from the island of Hispaniola, where the disease erupted in epidemic form, destroying about half of the population. From there the disease passed to Cuba and subsequently to Mexico, courtesy of an infected African slave in the party of the conquistador Panfilo de Narvaez, who was sent to meet with the party of Hernando Cortes.[89] Smallpox, the most virulent of the various pathogens imported by the Europeans, ravaged Amerindian societies to such an extent that when European forces pushed into the interior they often found villages filled with cadavers and devoid of survivors. This may partially account for the considerable military success that European forces enjoyed throughout their missions of conquest and subjugation. Crosby argues that smallpox was the pivotal variable providing for the socio-political destabilization of Amerindian societies, and their subsequent conquest by European forces.

The disease exterminated a large fraction of the Aztecs and cleared a path for the Spaniards to the heart of Tenochtitlan and to the founding of New Spain. Racing ahead of the conquistadores, it soon appeared in Peru, killing a large proportion of the subjects of the Inca, the Inca king, and the successor he had chosen. Civil war and chaos followed, and then Francisco Pizzaro arrived. The miraculous triumphs of that conquistador, and of Cortes, whom he so successfully emulated, are in large part the triumphs of the virus of smallpox.[90]

Estimates of the Amerindian population immediately before the arrival of the Europeans (in 1492) vary considerably. Russell Thornton has estimated the original population to have been circa 72 million in 1492, which was subsequently diminished by disease and war to a nadir of 600,000 in 1800.[91] Using the data of Henry Dobyns,[92] McNeil estimates that Amerindian societies declined from circa 28 million in 1520 to 3 million by 1568 and to approximately 1.6 million by 1620.[93] McNeill details the consequences of such demographic disaster: "Overall, the disaster to Amerindian populations assumed a scale that is hard for us to imagine. . . . Ratios of 20:1 or even 25:1 between pre-Columbian populations and the bottoming out (point). . . . Behind such cold statistics lurks enormous and repeated human anguish, as whole societies fell apart, values crumbled, and old ways of life lost all shred of meaning."[94] According to the historians James Lockhart and Serge Gruzinski, the Nahuatl population of Mexico Valley, which in 1518 supported an indigenous population of 25.2 million, had been reduced to 1.1 million by 1605.[95] The viral waves appear to be synchronous with political destabilization as the Aztec state imploded in 1521, the timing of which corresponds to the first waves of the virus.

The pox began to afflict the Inca in 1524, similarly resulting in the demographic collapse of the Andean population. The decline was evidently catastrophic, as the population base withered by 93 percent in the period 1524–1630.[96] The "pox" also resulted in the death of the Inca leader Huayna Capac, killed his heirs, disrupted succession, and ultimately facilitated Pizarro's conquests.[97] Such catastrophic and rapid declines in the population of a society generate profound psychological and social destabilization, and destroy the skill and knowledge base. Clearly, European military victories throughout the Americas were greatly facilitated by the pathogenic destruction of the antecedent populations and by the resultant collapse of their military power, erosion of elite legitimacy, and implosion of their structures of governance.[98] The pox also would seem to have influenced the outcome of the American Revolutionary War, during which the thirteen colonies of the nascent United States fought to secede from British rule. In this case the contagion was directly facilitated by the conditions of the war, but it also burned through the ranks of the forces on both sides and often incapacitated entire divisions. According to the historian Elizabeth Fenn, the destructive effects of the pox were exhibited during the campaign against Canada, wherein the American general Benedict Arnold watched as his forces were cut down by the pox during the siege of Quebec City in November of 1775.[99] As a result of the Canadian debacle, infectious disease became recognized as a significant threat to the integrity and efficacy of the US military, and thus perceived as a direct threat to national security.

Cholera

A water-borne illness induced by the bacterium *Vibrio cholerae*, cholera is now principally a disease of the indigent throughout the developing countries—a disease attributable to the lack of clean water and adequate sanitary infrastructure. Historically, however, cholera exhibited significant negative effects on prosperity and governance in the core states of Europe (particularly in regard to the evolution of health governance at the level of the state). It is thought to have caused the death of such philosophical and artistic luminaries as Hegel, Clausewitz,[100] and Tchaikovsky.[101] During the nineteenth century, cholera generated 130,000 deaths in the United Kingdom, while India lost approximately 25 million people to *Vibrio*.[102] Significant problems in the analysis of the historic impact of cholera emanate from the mortality data, as many who perished would have not been registered as victims of cholera, owing to the stigmatization of dying a "dog's death."[103] Further, until the German biologist Robert Koch identified the pathogen in 1884, there was no empirical means of accurate diagnosis. Thus, certain individuals who appeared to succumb to cholera may have in fact died of illnesses displaying similar symptoms (such as dysentery).[104]

The historian Richard Evans has argued that the novelty of the pathogen and its Eastern origins produced psychological trauma among afflicted European populations and undermined their assumptions of biological superiority. "All this," Evans writes, "made (cholera) into an object of peculiar terror and revulsion to the contemporary imagination, and further contributed to the shock effect it had on nineteenth-century society."[105] As the pathogen proliferated throughout Europe, the disease was viewed by the lower classes as a deliberate attempt by malign elites to poison them, fulfilling the Malthusian dictates of a draconian form of population control. As cholera swept across France in 1832, the historian Francois Delaporte notes, "the poor all over Europe shared the same fears and identified the same enemy, for the simple reason that cholera struck the poor first. People could not understand how a disease that attacked only the lower classes could be anything but intentional."[106] The uncertainty surrounding both the origins and vectors of transmission of cholera generated profound fear and anxiety, induced the perception and construction of elites as enemies, exacerbated mistrust between classes, and thereby augmented the potential for conflict between social factions. Such tensions often exploded into overt civil violence. Delaporte explains the "construction" of such a deliberate threat by the impassioned (and fearful) working class as a draconian solution to the problem of masses of poor, uneducated, and unproductive people.[107] The psychological demonization of "the other," and consequent manifestations of social tensions in the form of inter-class violence, often bedeviled European societies. The historian Frank Snowden shares these conclusions. "As at Naples in 1884," he writes, "cholera epidemics gave rise in many countries to serious social tensions, leading to riots, mass flight, and assaults on doctors and officials."[108]

Evans characterizes cholera's march across Europe during the 1830s as "marked by a string of riots and disturbances in almost every country it affected. Riots, massacres and the destruction of property took place across Russia, swept through the Hapsburg Empire, broke out in Königsberg, Stettin and Memel in 1831 and spread to Britain the next year."[109] Fear of contagion (and the poisoning hypothesis) led to pathos, to scapegoating of "the other," and to intra-state violence. According to Roderick McGrew, "the hysteria focused on particular scapegoats. The most popular villains were Polish agents and foreigners in general, though both physicians and government officials were also included. By midsummer a mass phobia had set in which affected the educated and the illiterate alike. . . . For the masses a spirit of evil had entered the land, and no one was immune. The poison scare played a part in the Petersburg cholera revolt, in the risings in the Novogorod military colonies, in the riots which occurred in Staraia Russia. . . ."[110]

Fearing massive disease-induced mortality and severe internal disruption, Czar Nicholas I adopted contagionist tactics, imposed a quarantine, and ordered that those infected be isolated. Such tactics failed to stem the spread of the pathogen and led to increasing social destabilization as the people reacted to the draconian measures of the state, with particularly serious riots in St. Petersburg in 1831.[111]

The British cholera epidemic of 1831 also incited riots, notably in Manchester. During the spring of that year, the public ascertained that the cadavers of cholera victims were being harvested by unscrupulous hospital authorities and sold to schools of anatomy. Furious citizens rose up in Manchester, among other cities, and demanded that their dead be treated with dignity.[112] Such riots in Britain were chronicled by the historian Michael Durey, who counted thirty cholera-induced riots in the United Kingdom between February and November 1832.[113] The appearance of cholera was also associated with the flight, or mass exodus, of citizens from affected regions, adding an additional dimension to the chaos that the illness generated. This phenomenon of contagion-induced refugees facilitated the expansion of the epidemic into naive populations.[114]

During this era, cholera infection also became associated with "immorality" (sex and drinking, specifically), providing the impetus for a legal crackdown by the state on such "unhealthy" habits.[115] As cholera-induced mortality mounted in Britain, the elites decided that segregation of the poor into "union houses" (also known as poorhouses) would be the most effective means of containing transmission. Parliament enacted the Poor Law Amendment Act of 1834, which entailed the creation of poorhouses based on parish. The conditions in these poorhouses were atrocious. According to Sheldon Watts, "the response of ordinary men and women was to dub the union poor-houses 'bastilles' and to keep clear of them. Within a generation, the idea that it was degrading, dishonorable, and depraved to allow oneself to be carted away to the poorhouse had become central to laboring people's system of values. The alternative—starvation or suicide at home—was seen as preferable."[116] Thus, cholera worsened the social stratification of British society and intensified the antipathy of one class toward the other. And through the closure of markets and the stagnation of business, not to mention the debilitation and/or destruction of human capital, cholera was instrumental in eroding the economic prosperity of affected regions.[117] After the international cholera control meetings held in Istanbul in 1866, trade was further constrained by London's imposition of exceptionally strict quarantine regulations on foreign vessels harboring infected persons.[118]

The extreme contagionist measures undermined citizens' perceptions of the legitimacy of state institutions and of certain elites associated with the state (namely physicians), and it promoted violence against ethnic groups who were seen as carriers.[119] Thus, acute social tensions and manifestations of violence were rampant during the first waves of epidemic cholera to strike Europe. Advances in public health and biology (courtesy of John Snow and Robert Koch) reduced uncertainty about the nature and source of the pathogen and about its vectors of transmission, and thereby resulted in a corresponding decline in fear and violence.

Yellow Fever

Yellow fever (caused by an arbovirus of the family *Flaviviridae* that induces hemorrhagic fevers)[120] has also had significant impacts on state-society relations, and at times on the trajectories of history. Such impacts range from a role in reinforcing the Jacobin coup and rebel government of former slaves in Haiti, to the Louisiana Purchase, to creating substantial problems of governance in the fledgling United States.

The breakdown in effective governance that resulted from the epidemic that struck Philadelphia in 1793 generated anxiety, panic, and even terror in the population. The contagion effectively closed down the federal government as Thomas Jefferson and George Washington fled the capital for the perceived safety of the countryside.[121] Alexander Hamilton, stricken by the illness, commented that "undue panic" was "fast depopulating the city, and suspending business both public and private."[122] Washington noted that even the heads of departments in the federal government would not carry out their duties, having discovered "matters of private concernment which required them to be absent."[123] Again, profound levels of negative affect accompanied the arrival of the contagion. According to the historian J. H. Powell, "people sickened of the fever, and they sickened of fear. Panic spread from heart to heart, fear paralyzed the whole as spasms racked the stricken, panic was the vicious ally of disease."[124]

The Philadelphia epidemic is an excellent example of the sclerotic (even paralytic) effects that contagion may induce within the institutions of the state. Indeed the epidemic of 1793 forced the early adjournment of Congress and the flight of legislators from the capitol, despite the apparent persistence of certain markets which remained open.[125] The disease-induced chaos that ensued confounded the effective operation of the federal government: "Public papers were locked up in closed houses when the clerks left. Postmaster-General Pickering and Attorney-General Randolph were off on an Indian treaty; their departments quickly fell apart, and they found nothing but confusion when they returned. President Washington had no one to inform him or bring him reports, none to advise or confer with him. The federal government had evaporated."[126]

Yellow fever was also associated with generating panic and the mass flight of individuals from affected areas. A classic example of such fear-induced exodus occurred during the New Orleans epidemic of May 1852, which caused more than 50,000 people to flee the city.[127] The fever resulted in 9,000 deaths, representing about 10 percent of New Orleans' citizens.[128] Once again the disease produced a sclerotic effect within the city, resulting in shutdowns of commerce and of basic government services.[129]

The fever was also instrumental in generating dislocation and socio-political chaos in Memphis, Tennessee in 1872. As the epidemic approached, economic elites fled the city, leaving behind a skeleton crew of municipal government officials who had enormous difficulty providing basic services to the frightened citizens. "After Autumn frosts put an end to the slaughter," Watts reports, "survivors met and petitioned that the bankrupt city find a new way to govern itself; the State obliged by canceling the city charter. While this was going on it was seriously suggested that the site of Memphis be abandoned, leveled to the ground and salted."[130]

On State-Society Relations

The Galenic tradition, its environmentalist precepts being derivative of Hippocrates, worked to undermine the discovery of the principle of contagion by the medical community during the 1400s. As Watts notes, it was during the 1450s that the political elites or "magistrates" of the cities of northern Italy discovered that infectious disease was in fact contagious.[131] The inability of medical "authorities" to contain disease, led to increasing disdain by the authorities (i.e., the state) for the Galenic[132] medical community, and thus one observes the rise of draconian controls by the state to suppress disease transmission.[133] Watts argues that centuries of persistent ineffectiveness of the medical community contributed to the widespread adoption of such hard-line positions by states in the sixteenth and seventeenth centuries:

The establishment of efficient quarantine control measures in port cities, of *cordon sanitaire* by armed troops and of information networks to warn of the approach of disease danger was all achieved by those European *civil authorities* who purposely ignored or overrode the objections of the medical doctors. By creating and enforcing the Ideology of Order in time of plague, princes considerably strengthened their hold over their subject populations. Quarantine procedures coincided with the gradual disappearance of plague from Western Europe: it last appeared in 1721.[134]

During periods of contagion, the historical record contains numerous instances of sovereign governments imposing significant (often draconian) controls on the behavior of the population, and on those who would enter the territory of the state. Such use of quarantine and martial law was termed "contagionist" and was typically associated with regimes that were held to be politically conservative. At the domestic level of analysis, then, the ascendancy of contagion worked to shift power away from civil society and toward the state. Contagionist thought was first articulated by Girolamo Fracastoro in his three-volume work *De contagione, contagiosis morbis et eorum curatione* (1546). Fracastoro argued that infectious agents generated human disease, and that epidemics were the resulting outcomes.[135] Containment measures enacted under the contagionist paradigm included military cordons of national boundaries, the identification and isolation of infected individuals, and the disinfection of trade goods and migrants. Despite its victories (depending on the pathogen in question) in containing the spread of epidemic disease, the paradigm is also historically associated with the intensification of political repression, as executed by the state against society in order to maintain the ideology of order, so popular with Central and Eastern European states of the time. Jean-Jacques Rousseau fell victim to the practices of quarantine and was detained at Genoa in 1743. His captivity, hunger, and frustration are detailed in his *Confessions*.[136] Given that contagionist philosophy emanated from the political elites of the time (primarily because of the persistent inadequacies of the Galenic community's response), it may correctly be seen as an effective implementation of social ingenuity in order to compensate for a lack of technical ingenuity.[137]

It is not my purpose here to re-open this age-old dispute between the contagionists and the environmental sanitationists,[138] but rather to discuss the impacts of epidemic disease on state and society, and the relationship between the two. The inherent peril associated with contagionism was that it held the potential for significant abuses of power by an unchecked bureaucracy, and that various manifestations of such abuses of society had in fact occurred over the centuries. For example, in Britain various waves of epidemic disease had resulted in the establishment of draconian policies of containment by the sovereign, including mandatory quarantines, lazarettos, the establishment of cordons and the execution of violators.[139] The popularity of contagionist thought spread beyond its European origins to become profoundly influential in Ottoman lands. Such externalization of contagionist thought became evident in 1840 when the Egyptian pasha Muhammad 'Ali, who ruled Egypt at the behest of the Ottoman Sultan, dismissed the opinions of his Galenic medical advisor. Based on contagionist successes in containing bubonic plague, Ali established the Florentine model of cordons and quarantine which effectively contained the pathogen in 1844.[140]

Despite the efficacy of contagionism in the containment of certain pathogens, the state's zeal in enforcing quarantinist measures often resulted in tensions between protection of the public good and the rights of the individual. Often such methods resulted in the erosion of the public's perceptions of the legitimacy of the state, and generated resistance (including violent riots) against the government.[141] Over the centuries, one can observe that the targets of popular aggression in times of epidemic shifted from minority groups toward the state and toward physicians who were seen to be allied with the government.[142] Evans notes the dynamics of such relations during the cholera years in Central Europe:

The coincidence of inexplicable outbreaks of mass mortality with the sudden appearance on the scene of government officials, troops, and medical officers readily aroused popular suspicion. It was not cholera by itself so much as the actions taken by the state against it which sparked off popular unrest. In Hungary, after over 1,000 cholera deaths between June and September 1831, castles were sacked and nobles massacred in an outburst of popular fury against those believed responsible for the deaths. In Russia military officers—themselves usually noble—bore the brunt of a good deal of popular hostility, as peasants attacked *cordons sanitaires* and murdered those who were trying to set them up.[143]

Those Prussian authorities who sought to contain epidemic disease using contagionist models often invoked national security concerns as a justification for their actions, and those who sought to evade the authorities were judged unpatriotic and even guilty of sedition.[144] But even as the state sought to protect its material interests from the destabilizing effects of disease, contagionist measures employed to stem the spread of disease subsequently imposed significant costs on the state as restrictions on markets and trade resulted in declining tax revenues.[145]

The balance of evidence as derived from the historical record suggests several preliminary conclusions regarding the validity of the postulates presented in the introduction. First, epidemic disease may generate widespread debilitation and/or significant levels of mortality within the population, which in turn often resulted in direct effects including the contraction of the economy and the depletion of state power. Further negative externalities emanated from the psychological "construction" of the epidemics by both state and society, often resulting in extreme societal tensions that occasionally took the form of riots and outright insurrection against the state. This "construction" of epidemics also generated societal instability through the stigmatization and persecution of the ill, manifestations of violence directed toward ethnic minorities and classes (elites), and the reinforcement of socio-economic inequities. Thus, visitations of infectious disease often presented the affected country with complex web of threats, both direct and indirect, that directly compromised the state's material interests and its base of power, and indirectly threatened the stability of the polity in its entirety. Second, in the domain of political science, there is increasing debate over whether health should be politicized, indeed "securitized." In recent years the debate has become sterile as those who recognize the potential threat that epidemics present to national security (what I shall refer to as the Florentine school)[146] and their ideological opposition (the Galenic school) talk past each other. This impasse is due largely to a lack of historical knowledge on the part of many of the protagonists on both sides, for, as we have seen, health has been associated with security concerns for centuries, indeed as far back as Thucydides. If we are to press ahead with improving our understanding of the links between health, prosperity, stability, and security, the Galenic school must acknowledge that issues of health have affected the calculus of power for sovereign countries, both internally and externally, for centuries. Finally, the Florentine School must recognize the perils arising from potential abuses of power by the sovereign state against its own citizens, in the name of maintaining order in the face of contagion, and must guard against such egregious abuses.

3

Pandemic Influenza: On Sclerosis in Governance

The unprecedented ferocity of World War I (1914–1918) saw the great powers of Europe galvanize their populations into "total war" and the Continent besieged by violence, chaos, and destruction. Ultimately, the conflict resulted in the disintegration of several empires; witness the centrifugal fragmentation of Austria-Hungary, the dissolution of the Ottoman Empire, and the subjugation of Germany under the punitive Treaty of Versailles.[1] The Great War, as it was also known, cut down a generation of young men in Europe and directly contributed to the emergence of a deadly influenza pandemic, known at the time as the Spanish Flu. The manifestations of pandemic influenza were horrific. Infected individuals exhibited heliotrope cyanosis, a bluish discoloration of the skin resulting from suffocation as their lungs filled with blood and fluid. The end result for the host was often systemic hemorrhaging, and ultimately death.

I begin this chapter by examining the impact of the 1918 pandemic on the institutions of affected sovereign states, their societies, and the interface between the two. A comparative demographic analysis of available mortality and morbidity data is followed by a description of the peculiar etiology of the 1918 pathogen. I then explore the effects of the pandemic on the state, and in particular its effect on the military forces (and societies) of the various protagonists in World War I, primarily through the available German, Austrian, British, French, and American data. Following that, I analyze the effects of the pandemic on governance (broadly construed) in affected polities.

Demographic Impact

During the final year of the Great War, pandemic influenza affected and debilitated circa 25 percent of the global population, typically resulting in the mortality of between 2 and 4 percent of those afflicted. Death typically resulted from influenza-induced hemorrhaging or suffocation, or from secondary pneumonic or tubercular co-infections.[2] In the United States, flu-induced morbidity was circa 25 million, with an estimated mortality of 675,000. According to the medical historian Hans Zinsser, the epidemic exerted a dramatic (if rather brief) negative effect on average US life expectancy, resulting in a significant decline of 12 years in 1918.[3]

"The pandemic," Alfred Crosby concludes,

affected history in general in the way that the random addition of a poison to some of the refreshments served at the 1918 West Point commencement celebrations would have affected the military history of World War II; i.e. it had enormous influence but one that utterly evades logical analysis and that has been completely ignored by all commentators on the past. On the level of organizations and institutions—the level of collectivities—the Spanish flu had little impact. It did not spur great changes in the structure and procedures of governments, armies, corporations, or universities. It had little influence on the course of political and military struggles because it usually affected all sides equally.[4]

Crosby's argument is based on a reading of US mortality data; however, the data presented below indicate that the pandemic did *not* affect all the protagonists equally. The balance of evidence indicates that the virus generated differential mortality across the spectrum of affected societies. The very fact that mortality varied so greatly across cultures leads to the conclusion that the pandemic had differential impacts on the various combatants involved in the war. A second point is that there was considerable temporal variation in the waves of pandemic influenza that circulated the world in 1918–19, and that it struck and debilitated the Central Powers before it struck the Allies.

The first evidence to challenge Crosby's assertion that all sides were affected equally by the pathogen comes from the medical historian W. H. Frost, who used the rates of mortality in mid-size to large population centers to document the degree to which influenza swept the United States in 1918. Importantly, Frost's data clearly indicate differential rates of morbidity across US population centers, ranging from 15 percent in Louisville to 53 percent in San Antonio.[5] Reinforcing this finding that flu-induced mortality was not uniform, but rather ranged along a continuum within societies, the medical historian Edgar Sydenstricker estimated that US national mortality rates ranged from 2.76 percent to

4.6 percent.[6] Considering this estimate in terms of rates, Crosby noted that (according to US Public Health Service surveys conducted at the time) 280 per thousand US citizens contracted pandemic influenza in 1918–19. Crosby extrapolates to conclude that over 25 percent of the US population was infected and debilitated by the contagion.[7]

Given that influenza-induced morbidity and mortality appears to have ranged along a continuum within societies, one might expect to observe considerable variance between sovereign states. The data bear out this supposition, as certain countries (e.g., Japan) exhibited exceptionally low mortality rates, whereas other countries exhibited exceptional to catastrophic levels of mortality (the worst case being Samoa). The medical demographers G. Rice and E. Palmer analyzed Japanese medical archives to compile data on influenza-related morbidity and mortality, and determined that Japan witnessed 2,168,398 cases (morbidity) and 257,363 deaths (mortality). "The case rate," they write, "was therefore 370 per thousand, or just over one-third of the whole population, which was rather higher than that of the United States. However, the influenza-induced crude death rate was rather minute, at 4.5 per thousand."[8] Other societies were not so fortunate. Data collected by Colin Brown indicate that Indonesia's mortality rate was approximately 17.7 per thousand.[9] Furthermore, approximately 3 percent of Sierra Leone's indigenous population died as a direct result of influenza by late 1918,[10] and Patterson has established that flu-induced mortality in African societies ranged from 30 to 40 per thousand.[11]

Attempts to quarantine Australia and New Zealand were partially successful; they only delayed the onset of the contagion, and Rice notes that New Zealand's Maori population exhibited a mortality rate of 43 per thousand.[12] Mills has established that India suffered to an even greater extent from the virus, with a mortality rate ranging from 46 to 67 per thousand, again varying by region.[13] The highest death rates appear to have occurred among the isolated and immunologically naive populations of islands such as Western Samoa, which exhibited a staggering mortality rate of 220 per thousand, resulting in the destruction of over 20 percent of its population base over the duration of the pandemic.[14] (See figure 3.1.)

Initial estimates of deaths induced by pandemic influenza placed aggregate global mortality at circa 21 million. However, recent epidemiological investigations have revealed that flu-induced mortality in South Asia

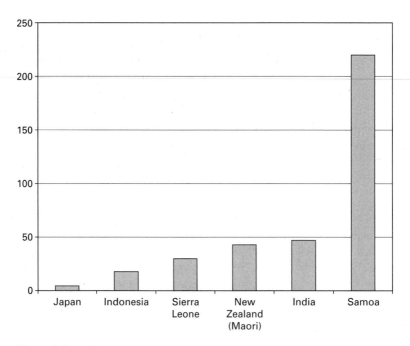

Figure 3.1
Influenza: comparative crude death rate per thousand, 1918–19.

alone (particularly in India) exceeded 17 million. Therefore, conservative revised estimates of mortality currently approach 50 million,[15] and liberal estimates are as high as circa 100 million.[16] For the purposes of this inquiry it seems prudent to adopt the figure of 50 million.

During typical manifestations of the pathogen, influenza is a killer of those at the two tails of the demographic distribution of a society: the very young and the elderly. Yet the 1918 epidemic displayed an unusual penchant for the destruction of healthy and productive individuals in the prime of their lives. Specifically, during the 1918 pandemic, the mortality distribution associated with infection exhibited the form of a W, with pronounced mortality in the 15–45-year age range, accompanied by the expected high mortality in the elderly and young.[17] Flu-induced mortality seems to have affected females and males in equal fashion, although the pathogen apparently generated exceptional mortality in pregnant mothers.[18] Why would the pathogen affect so many healthy young adults in the prime of their lives? It is reasonable to speculate that the influenza generated a profound overreaction by the body's immune system, and that the cytokines (endogenous toxins) released by the body destroyed the fragile tissues of the lungs during the immune system's attempt to combat the virus.[19] It would seem, then, that those with stronger immune systems were, as a perverse consequence, more vulnerable to the pathogen.

Beyond the influenza, various pathogens exhibited a pronounced and deleterious effect on the German population during World War I. One reasonable explanation for such declines in German public health is that the embargo on the shipment of foodstuffs to the Central Powers during this period would have severely compromised the base health of the average German citizen, increasing the probability of colonization of the human host by the pathogen. Indeed, male civilian deaths in Germany peaked in 1918 at 566,077, with female mortality in the same year reaching a zenith of 644,163 even though females were non-combatants. Compare such figures with postwar baseline civilian mortality of 429,741 for males and 426,263 for females in the year 1923.[20] Note that this post-conflict baseline may be rather inflated relative to prewar data, owing to the fact that the war generated attenuated negative impacts on human health, ranging from immunosuppression and secondary infection to mental illness.[21]

Etiology

Recent evidence suggests that the 1918 influenza was in fact an H1N1 variant, and therefore genetically similar to the virus currently spreading throughout avian populations in East and Southeast Asia. The 1918 virus likely originated in avian species, crossed over into the human ecology through processes of zoonotic transmission, then continued to evolve and mutate within human populations. This helps to account for the three waves of the pandemic that circled the world in 1918, each progressively more lethal, and likely intensified by the conditions of World War I.

The orthodox epidemiological history traces the origins of the pandemic to Camp Funston (near Fort Riley, in Kansas) during March 1918, after which it appeared at Camp Oglethorpe in Georgia and then at Camp Devens in Massachusetts.[22] With troop transport vessels serving as vectors of both incubation and distribution, the flu then supposedly traveled to the battlefields of Europe, whereupon it infected thousands of soldiers during the spring of 1918. During this initial phase, the pathogen exhibited significant morbidity, with slightly elevated mortality, and then entered a period of relative dormancy during the summer months that followed. Late August of 1918 saw the second wave of the epidemic erupt with much greater lethality, appearing simultaneously in France, Sierra Leone, and the United States (with its epicenter in Boston).

The third and most virulent wave of the epidemic appeared in the fall of 1918, attacking the military forces of both the United States and the Central Powers and overwhelming field hospitals, transports, and lazarets in the rear with fevered, debilitated, and dying young men. According to the microbiologist Paul Ewald, throughout these three increasingly lethal waves of infection, the influenza virus progressively mutated to take advantage of the densely packed populations and of the mobility of soldiers, resulting in the emergence of a highly communicable and lethal strain. Ewald notes that the mobility of forces acted as a "cultural vector" to distribute the virus from infected host populations to uninfected populations:

Soldiers in the trenches were grouped so closely that even immobile infecteds could transmit pathogens. When a soldier was too sick to fight, he was typically removed by his trenchmates. But by that time trenchmates often would have been infected.[23]

Thus, the malign ecological conditions associated with a protracted ground war allowed the virus to mutate in order to become more infective (and increasingly lethal) to the young adult populations that served as hosts in the theater of war, and resulting in the unusual W-shaped mortality distribution. Ewald writes:

The increased mortality in the trenches due to fighting or the other infectious diseases that typically accompanied such warfare should have, if anything, also favored a high level of virulence. Any deaths of recovered immune individuals would result in the transport of replacements into the trenches who would often be susceptible to the strains circulating in the trenches. In addition, one of the costs that a pathogen may incur from extremely rapid reproduction is a shortened duration of infection due either to a more rapid immune response or to host death.[24]

Thus, the epidemic was a product of the pernicious ecology of war, with high population densities of combatants, poor sanitation, stress, and the movement of forces collectively serving as remarkably efficient vectors of transmission around the world. However, the pandemic may have also affected the course of the war, to some degree, through its successive waves of debilitation and destruction of human life. Thus, we may understand the relationship between war, pathogenic emergence, and outcome of the war as a complex feedback mechanism. I shall explore this concept in greater detail below.

On the Political Suppression of Data

The effects of the contagion were historically downplayed by the medical community, who (like the Galenists of old) were acutely embarrassed by their impotence in the face of such an overwhelming epidemic. According to the medical historian Carol Byerly, "the tendency of medical officers, army commanders, and federal officials to downplay the role of the influenza epidemic in the Great War, and the impact of disease on military populations in general, has encouraged American complacency about the ability of medicine to control disease outbreaks during war."[25] The German medical historian Wilfried Witte has noted that Prussian authorities went out of their way to downplay the severity of the pandemic during wartime, going so far as to repress the dissemination of data as best they could. Furthermore, existing data suggest that, while the majority of deaths were recorded in urban centers, there was significant debilitation and mortality in rural areas that likely went unrecorded because of a lack of medical personnel in those regions. Therefore, many of the mortality data from Central Europe are probably significantly lower than the actual mortality that occurred as a result of both repression and low levels of health-care capacity in rural regions.[26] Johnson and Mueller concur with the assessment that available estimates vastly understate the impact of the contagion on mortality. They posit that "limitations of these data can include nonregistration, missing records, misdiagnosis, and nonmedical certification, and may also vary greatly between locations."[27]

The general dearth of investigation regarding the political and economic effects of the Spanish Flu are notable, and necessarily raise some questions. "The influenza epidemic's most important, if enigmatic, legacy," Byerly argues, "has been its reinforcement of the government's and the society's reluctance to acknowledge the deadly role disease often plays in war. As people have written war stories and official reports of wars, they have often effaced human suffering, reflecting the military's tendency to downplay the fact of injury as a product of war. This tendency is especially apparent with respect to the story of disease in war."[28]

Because death from disease was often regarded as ignoble, in the aftermath of the Great War military forces sought to diminish the perceived impact of the contagion, particularly since military medical officers had been utterly powerless in the face of such a pathogen. Byerly castigates the US government for its deliberate and widespread attempts to suppress evidence of mortality from disease during the conflict. She argues that the War Department's official record of the war "listed battle casualties only" and that "a 1919 Senate document on the cost of the war stated that 50,000 men were killed in battle. Although this report calculated various costs of the war . . . it failed to mention the war cost of 57,000 deaths from disease. It reduced the army death toll by more than half."[29]

Effects on the State

Central to this analysis is the effect of pathogens on the apparatus of governance within a polity, particularly the bureaucracy and the military.

The profound morbidity and mortality induced by the pandemic affected the armed forces of the various combatants in different fashions. Much as countries exhibited differential mortality from the contagion, the armed forces of states exhibited varying death rates. Comparative analyses of the causes of death for military forces, measuring mortality from disease versus that suffered in action, are illustrative. On the Allied side, US forces experienced the most severe impacts of the contagion, with a rough 1:1 ratio of deaths from disease to battlefield injuries.[30] French forces saw a much lower mortality ratio (roughly 1:6), and in British forces the ratio was approximately 1:10.[31] Such variance in mortality contradicts Crosby's postulate that all the belligerents were affected to the same degree by the pandemic. It also demonstrates that the British and French forces may have had more acquired immunity to the pathogen than their American counterparts.

Aside from the direct costs imposed by troop mortality, the effects of the influenza on military personnel included debilitation, decline of morale, and the diversion of the leadership's focus from the prosecution of the war to containment of the contagion. Additionally, the death and debilitation of officers undermined force cohesion, planning, and execution, and reduced the capacity for effective reinforcement of divisions in the midst of battle. It also diminished the military's capacity for the medical evacuation of ill personnel to hospitals, where health providers also succumbed to the virus. Thus, although the contagion did not utterly paralyze the machinery of war, it did slow military units down, notably diminishing their efficacy.

The United States

During the supposed first wave of pandemic influenza that appeared in the United States during the spring of 1918, initial mortality in military training facilities hovered around 10 per thousand. Such mortality eventually declined to mere 2.3 per thousand by mid September of 1918.[32] However, the most virulent strain arrived soon after that point, and on October 11, 1918, mortality soared to 206 per thousand.[33] The morbidity and mortality associated with the pandemic had profoundly deleterious consequences for the operational capacity of many US military units. In September 1918, US Brigadier General Charles Richard commented to his peers: "Epidemic influenza . . . has become a very serious menace and threatens not only to retard the military program, but to exact a heavy toll in human life. . . ."[34] In the US experience, pandemic influenza induced absenteeism, loss of morale, and logistical chaos throughout the military infrastructure. The historian James Seidule argues that influenza had a significant negative effect on the morale of US forces and undermined their logistical cohesion during the conflict: "The flu sapped the strength and the morale of everyone in the AEF [and it] combined with malnutrition, inadequate clothing, and lack of sleep to create thousands of soldiers who suffered from combat exhaustion. . . . The result was an ineffective army with low morale."[35] Crosby describes the effects of the contagion on the US 57th Pioneer Infantry during their march to the naval vessels that would ferry them to France: "Some men stayed where they had sprawled. Others, almost as sick, struggled to their feet to keep up with their platoons, even throwing away equipment to avoid falling behind. No one was ever able to determine how much equipment or how many men the 57th lost on that march."[36]

The rise of influenza had other pernicious effects on the war-fighting capacity of US forces, including logistical problems and the quarantine of US training camps. Eventually the virus resulted in suspension of the draft: "On September 26, with Pershing calling for reinforcements, with the AEF (American Expeditionary Force) pushing forward into the Argonne . . . the Provost Marshal General of the United States Army canceled an October draft call for 142,000 men. Practically all the camps to which they had been ordered were quarantined. The call up of 78,000 additional men in October had to be postponed. . . ."[37] Crosby notes that the strains of the pandemic forced a 10 percent reduction in troop shipments to France. Furthermore, on October 11, 1918, "the War Department ordered a reduction in the intensity of training at all army camps. At the end of the month, the Chief of Staff in Washington wired General Pershing that the flu had stopped nearly all draft calls and practically all training in October."[38]

The pandemic thereby undermined the American Expeditionary Force's prosecution of the Meuse-Argonne Offensive, which began on September 26 and concluded on November 11, 1918. "When Pershing needed 90,000 replacement troops for his Meuse-Argonne campaign," Byerly argues, [US Army Chief of Staff] March could provide him with only 45,000 because of the epidemic."[39] Indeed, during the Meuse-Argonne offensive, the estimated US morbidity from influenza was 68,760, as compared to 69,832 soldiers wounded by bullets and 18,864 who succumbed to gas.[40] The comparative mortality statistics of the US 88th division are also illustrative regarding the effects of the pandemic. "The total of all combat losses for the 88th—killed, wounded, missing, and captured—was 90. The total of its flu cases during the fall wave was 6,845 [or] approximately one-third of the division. One thousand and forty five contracted pneumonia, and 444 died."[41]

Alexander Stark, chief surgeon of the First Army, concluded that "influenza so clogged the medical services and the evacuation system, and rendered 'ineffective' so many men in the armies that it threatened to disrupt the war."[42] "By the War Department's own account," according to Byerly, "flu sickened 26 percent of the army—more than one million men—and accounted for 82 percent of total deaths from disease."[43]

Given the malign synergy between the influenza virus and secondary sources of infection, one must include much of the subsequent mortality from infections (after October 1918) within the aggregate assessment of pandemic-induced mortality. Comprehensive assessments of mortality by the US War Department showed that the contagion actually killed more American troops than deaths from injuries sustained in combat. Specifically, while 50,280 American soldiers were killed in action, 57,460 died from pandemic influenza.[44] The US War Department eventually estimated that the pandemic resulted in the loss of 8,743,102 person-days to influenza among enlisted personnel in 1918 alone.[45] The US Navy was particularly affected by the destructive capacity of the pathogen: "All in

all, the US Navy lost 4,136 of its officers and men to the flu and pneumonia in the last third of 1918. Despite the efforts of Germany's under-
sea fleet, almost twice as many Americans soldiers died in the pandemic
than as the result of enemy action in 1918."[46] US Naval statistics compiled during the course of the contagion indicate that circa 40 percent
of naval personnel succumbed to the flu during 1918. Meanwhile, 361
per 1,000 US soldiers were admitted to hospital in 1918 for complica-
tions arising from influenza infection. "In total over 621,000 [US] soldiers caught the flu in 1918, upwards of one-sixth of the total number
of American soldiers in World War I."[47] Furthermore, assessments of
morbidity provide an indication of the aggregate impact of influenza on
military effectiveness. The records of the Surgeon General of the US
Army indicate that, of the 1 million men of the AEF who were hospitalized, circa 775,000 were hospitalized because of illness (influenza), while
the remaining 225,000 were hospitalized for wounds incurred on the
battlefield.[48] Additional data indicate that 26 percent of the personnel in
Army units were similarly debilitated by the pathogen.[49]

In the final analysis, US War Department records indicate that morbidity associated with the conflict saw 227,000 hospitalized for wounds
incurred in battle, while over 340,000 were hospitalized for influenza.[50]
According to War Department records, the Army Surgeon General noted
that debilitation and death from influenza had resulted in the loss of
9,055,659 days of manpower, with the result that almost two full divisions were out of action for the entire year 1918.[51]

Britain and France

According to Byerly, the influenza pandemic induced approximately
225,000 deaths among civilians in the United Kingdom.[52] The British
Expeditionary Forces saw approximately 313,000 cases (morbidity) of
influenza during 1918, although incomplete records suggest that this
estimate may be on the conservative side.[53]

Current estimates of French civilian flu-induced mortality are approximately 135,000, and France lost circa 30,000 soldiers to the virus over
the course of the pandemic.[54] Crosby argues that, in September 1918
alone, French forces in the combat zone exhibited over 25,000 cases of
influenza, and that "the rear-area soldiers, not the men in actual combat,
bore the brunt of the pandemic. The incidence of Flu in the French Army
in the interior areas, for instance, was three to twelve times higher than
in the French army at or near the battlefront."[55] This suggests that the

rear camps may have acted as optimal vectors of viral dissemination, superior to transmission within the trenches.

Furthermore, the three waves of influenza that swept over the United Kingdom saw three distinct mortality peaks. The first peak occurred from July 6 to 14, 1918, the second from October 19 to November 23, 1918, and the third from February 8 to March 15, 1919.[56] It is extremely significant to note that the waves of mortality that swept through Allied forces were not synchronous with those waves of mortality that swept across the citizens (and military forces) of the Central European states. The temporal variability of the mortality waves, hitting the Central Powers first, helps to further dispel the assertion that the influenza affected all the combatants in a roughly equivalent manner. As the German and Austrian data cited below indicate , the waves of mortality visited on those societies significantly preceded those that swept the United Kingdom, with possibly significant historical consequences.

Germany

The emergence of the virulent form of the contagion in the spring of 1918 coincided with the German Offensive of the Somme. During this period, the German Chief of Staff, General Erich Von Ludendorff, complained vociferously about the deleterious effects of the influenza on German military efficacy. The Somme offensive, which began on March 21, 1918, began to sputter in May as the virus increasingly debilitated German troops and crippled their units. In late June of that year, Ludendorff "noted that over 2000 men in each division were suffering from influenza, that the supply system was breaking down, and that troops were underfed. Infection spread rapidly. By late July, Ludendorff specifically blamed the pandemic for nullifying the German drive."[57] According to the historian Richard Bessel, "the influenza outbreaks in among the (German) troops in June and July 1918, left very great numbers of sick and wounded in their wake: of the 1.4 million German soldiers who participated in the offensives, over 300,000 became casualties between 21 March and 10 April, and the influenza epidemic in June and July alone affected more than half a million men; altogether between March and July 1918 about 1.75 million German soldiers fell ill at some point and roughly 750,000 were wounded."[58] Empirical data confirm Bessel's assertions and Ludendorff's protestations. Figure 3.2 illustrates the profound (and non-linear) increase in flu-induced mortality in the German Army. The pathogen-induced destruction was so profound, and the

German physicians and nurses so overwhelmed by the dead and dying, that they were unable to keep track of the mortality as the first wave of the pandemic struck in the early days of June 1918, with over 15 percent of forces infected before the physicians were overwhelmed and ceased to register incidence.

Aside from the direct effects of mortality and morbidity, the flu also undermined the logistical efficacy of the German military: it adversely affected the effective function of the railways throughout the late summer and fall of 1918, impeding the timely distribution of materiel.[59] "Influenza," Crosby observes, "gummed up the German supply lines and made it harder to advance and harder to retreat. From the point of view of the generals, it had a worse effect on the fighting qualities of an army than death itself. The dead were dead. . . . But the flu took good men and made them into delirious staggering debits whose care required the diversion of healthy men from important tasks."[60]

Ludendorff continued to lament the contagion's pernicious effects on the German military effort. "Our army suffered," he wrote. "Influenza was rampant. . . . It was a grievous business having to listen every morning to the chiefs of staffs' recital of the number of influenza cases, and their complaints about the weakness of their troops if the English attacked again."[61] The death and debilitation arising from the pandemic also appear to have affected discipline and morale among German forces.[62] According to Crosby, Ludendorff later "blamed the failure of his July offensive, which came so close to winning the war for Germany, on the poor morale and diminished strength of his armies, which he attributed in part to flu."[63]

The public health records of the German military indicate that their forces were burdened by circa 1,543,612 cases of lethal influenza (then called "the Grippe"). Morbidity among German troops increased from a rate of 131,139 cases per annum in 1914 to 896,266 per annum in 1918,[64] an increase of 683.18 percent over the course of the war.

According to the medical historian Fielding Garrison, infection rates ranged from 16 percent to 80 percent of soldiers, depending on the unit.[65] By October 17, influenza had thoroughly debilitated the German forces and was raging all along the front. Bessel argues that the final lethal wave of influenza in October 1918 may have contributed to the ultimate collapse of the German war effort, and to the decline in effective governance by the state:

Krankenzugang an Grippe (Rapp. Nr. 8) bei den Truppen

Übersicht 105.

1. ——— des Deutschen Feldheeres, 2. – – – – des Deutschen Besatzungsheeres, 3. ...... der Preuß. usw. Armee im Durchschnitt 1907/12, berechnet auf 1000 Mann der durchschnittlichen Iststärke.

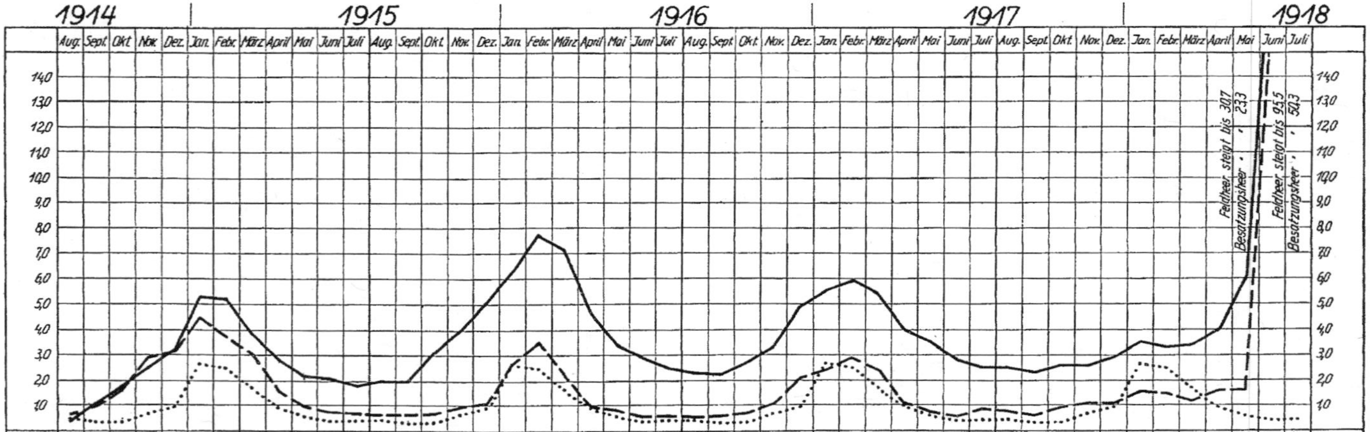

1914	Aug.	Sept.	Okt.	Nov.	Dez.
Feldheer ———	0,37	1,1	1,8	2,5	3,2
Besatzungsheer – – –	0,63	0,98	1,7	2,9	3,2
Preuß. usw. Arm. 1907/8+1911/12	0,45	0,34	0,35	0,70	0,93

1915	Jan.	Febr.	März	April	Mai	Juni	Juli	Aug.	Sept.	Okt.	Nov.	Dez.
Feldheer ———	5,3	5,2	3,8	2,8	2,2	2,1	1,8	2,0	2,0	3,1	4,0	5,1
Besatzungsheer – – –	4,5	3,7	3,0	1,6	0,97	0,74	0,69	0,67	0,68	0,70	0,95	1,1
Preuß. usw. Arm. 1907/8+1911/12	2,7	2,5	1,7	0,93	0,60	0,41	0,42	0,45	0,34	0,35	0,70	0,93

1916	Jan.	Febr.	März	April	Mai	Juni	Juli	Aug.	Sept.	Okt.	Nov.	Dez.
Feldheer ———	6,3	7,7	7,1	4,7	3,4	2,9	2,5	2,3	2,2	2,7	3,4	4,9
Besatzungsheer – – –	2,7	3,5	2,2	0,98	0,81	0,60	0,61	0,59	0,62	0,72	1,1	2,1
Preuß. usw. Arm. 1907/8+1911/12	2,7	2,5	1,7	0,93	0,60	0,41	0,42	0,45	0,34	0,35	0,70	0,93

1917	Jan.	Febr.	März	April	Mai	Juni	Juli	Aug.	Sept.	Okt.	Nov.	Dez.
Feldheer ———	5,5	5,9	5,4	4,0	3,5	2,8	2,5	2,5	2,3	2,6	2,6	2,9
Besatzungsheer – – –	2,4	2,9	2,4	1,1	0,73	0,58	0,88	0,78	0,62	0,91	1,1	1,1
Preuß. usw. Arm. 1907/8+1911/12	2,7	2,5	1,7	0,93	0,60	0,41	0,42	0,45	0,34	0,35	0,70	0,93

1918	Jan.	Febr.	März	April	Mai	Juni	Juli
Feldheer ———	3,5	3,3	3,4	4,0	6,0	30,7	95,5
Besatzungsheer – – –	1,6	1,5	1,2	1,6	1,6	23,3	50,3
Preuß. usw. Arm. 1907/8+1911/12	2,7	2,5	1,7	0,93	0,60	0,41	0,42

Übersicht 106.   Die Grippeerkrankungen bei der Truppe

Zeitraum	des Besatzungsheeres	des Feldheeres				
		im ganzen	an der Westfront	an der Ostfront	auf dem Balkan	in der Türkei
von August 1917 bis Mai 1918	24 675	170 254	184 271	31 076	2 467	485
⁰/₀₀ G.	1,2	3,3	3,8	2,9	2,4	4,1
im Juni 1918	51 071	138 781	135 002	3 298	435	51
⁰/₀₀ G.	23,3	30,6	35,1	5,3	8,2	6,2
im Juli 1918	112 214	399 271	374 524	21 747	2 995	?
⁰/₀₀ G.	50,3	94,5	104,4	36,9	57,8	?

Übersicht 107.   Der Zugang an Grippe von der Truppe in die Lazarette betrug

Zeitraum	beim Feldheer	beim Besatzungsheer
von August 1917 bis Mai 1918	43 990	9 786
im Juni 1918	27 867	10 208
im Juli 1918	52 542	26 604

Figure 3.2

Influenza mortality, German armed forces, 1917–1919. Source: *Sanitätsbericht über das deutsche Heer im Weltkriege 1914/1918,* volume 3 (Mittler & Sohn, 1934).

... in the last months of 1918 the military demobilization coincided with a sharp increase in mortality caused by the influenza epidemic: German civilian deaths shot up in October 1918 (when they were nearly two and a half times what they had been in September), remained extremely high in November, and returned to average wartime levels only in March 1919. Indeed, the months of October and November 1918 registered the highest civilian mortality rates in Germany for the entire war.[66]

With the notable exceptions of Bessel and Crosby, there has been a tendency among historians to discount Ludendorff's accounts of the flu as given to wild exaggeration and exhibiting a tendency to deny accountability. However, Ludendorff's accounts of the influenza are very much supported by empirical data culled from the Prussian State archives of the Staatsbibliothek in Berlin. (See figure 3.3.)

Waves of subsequent mortality due to secondary infection resulted from the destruction that the influenza had wreaked on its human hosts' immune systems, particularly on the fragile tissues of the lungs. The most prevalent of these post-flu infections was tuberculosis, which claimed the lives of 40,043 German women in 1914 and 66,608 in 1918. Similarly, German female deaths resulting from pneumonia rose from 35,700 in 1914 to 74,468 in 1918.[67] Collectively, this indicates that the conditions associated with the war resulted in increases of German female mortality of 66.34 percent for tuberculosis and 208.59 percent for pneumonia, both of which were typical post-flu secondary infections. Not only did the contagion kill productive members of German society and contribute to post-hoc infections and mortality; it also resulted in the profound and attenuated debilitation of survivors, to the extent that it undermined the productivity of the German workforce, and hence the German war effort, from the spring of 1918 to the collapse of the government in November of that year.[68] Additional evidence for this drop in productivity comes from the dramatic declines in German coal production caused by influenza, as noted in the records of mines from that period.[69] Such steep declines in the pivotal energy resource of the time would have had a profound negative effect on the capacity of the German military in particular, and on the resilience of the macro economy in general. Bessel has also noted that the rise of the influenza pandemic temporally coincides with the failure of the German military effort, the collapse of effective governance, and the advent of revolution.[70] The data on morbidity and mortality support such assertions to a degree.

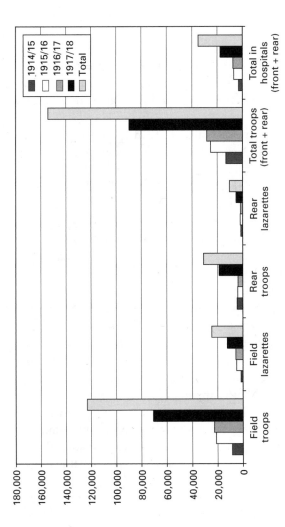

Figure 3.3
Influenza morbidity, German armed forces, 1914–1918. Source: *Sanitätsbericht über das deutsche heer im Weltkriege 1914/1918*, volume 3 (Mittler & Sohn, 1934).

Austria-Hungary

The pandemic visited considerable suffering and destruction on the Central Powers and, as the data cited in figure 3.4 indicate, may have also resulted in limiting the martial power and the stable governance of Austria-Hungary.

The Austrian data (rather more complete than the German records) indicate that influenza struck Austria-Hungary in a single dramatic wave during late October and early November of 1918, whereas the rest of the world apparently suffered through three waves of influenza, beginning in the spring of 1918, each more lethal than the last. The Austrians apparently only suffered the visitation of the last and deadliest viral wave, which cut through the population in late October 1918.

The data suggest that the Austrians witnessed a previously unacknowledged regional epidemic of considerable influenza-induced mortality during the first and second quarters of 1917, significantly predating the viral waves that began in the spring of 1918 in the United States. This revelation suggests that a precursor epidemic, of unknown origins, apparently swept through Austria (and perhaps other regions of Central Europe) in the spring of 1917. This provides empirical evidence to reinforce John Oxford's hypothesis that the virus may have emerged in sporadic epidemic form before 1918.[71] What is apparent in the Viennese case is that the Austrian people did not experience the two increasingly lethal waves of pandemic influenza that swept the world in the spring and summer of 1918 but suffered a lingering pandemic. From an epidemiological viewpoint, the lack of exposure to these two waves in early 1918 may have inhibited the Austrian population's development of any significant immunity to the final genetic variant of the pathogen, thereby increasing their vulnerability to the third wave.

Such empirical evidence of a Austrian precursor epidemic that generated significant mortality in the spring of 1917 is of profound epidemiological significance. It explains how the Austrians may have developed partial immunity to the viral waves of spring and summer 1918, as a direct result of that prior exposure. However, they apparently remained immunologically naive to the genetically novel and exceptionally lethal variant of the virus that appeared in the fall of 1918 and generated such enormous mortality in the fourth quarter of that year.

Further, one must recall the pathogenic connectivity between influenza, which destroyed the hosts lungs and immune system, and the opportunistic infections (such as viral and bacterial pneumonia) that then

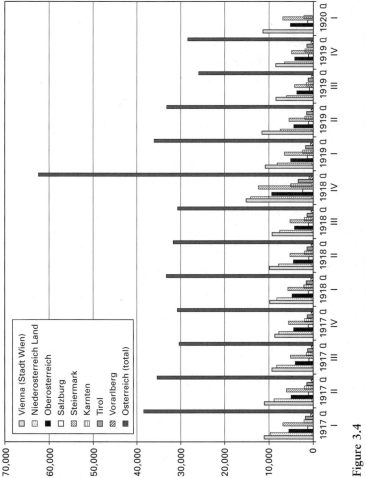

Figure 3.4
Influenza mortality, Austria, 1917–1919, by quarter. Source: Siegfried Rosenfeld, *Die Grippeepidemie das Jahres 1918 im Österreich* (Volksgesundheitsamte im Bundesministerium für Soziale Verwaltung, 1921).

debilitated and often killed the weakened host. Additional data from Austria indicate that the influenza pandemic generated a subsequent wave of pneumonic mortality throughout the Austrian people. This secondary wave of infection significantly augmented the mortality generated by the final viral wave of influenza. Furthermore, it is interesting to note that an earlier peak in pneumonia-induced mortality appears to be synchronous with the observed "first wave" of influenza mortality that struck Austria in the spring of 1917.[72] (See figure 3.5.)

The historical record indicates that the final viral wave of influenza (and the nigh synchronous wave of deaths from pneumonia) immediately preceded the fragmentation of the Empire. Specifically, within two weeks of the final wave of the virus' striking Vienna, the Austro-Hungarian Empire underwent utter political disintegration. Thus, mortality from the "third wave" constituted an exogenous shock of some magnitude, and one that may have served as the proverbial "straw that broke the camel's back." It is quite certain that influenza was not the sole agent responsible for the dissolution of the empire. However, the influenza pandemic undoubtedly functioned as a powerful stressor to shatter the rotten and tottering foundations of the institutions of the empire, which had been successively eroded by years of war.

Pandemic Influenza's Impact on World War I

With the notable exceptions of Crosby, Byerly, and Bessel, medical historians have perpetuated the ignorance of the impact of influenza on the war effort, and certainly on the outcome of the war. The historians Byron Farwell, Jennifer Keene, and Robert Ziegler have argued that the pandemic compromised the effectiveness of military forces during the war to a certain extent, but they have not gone so far as to argue that it had any effect on the outcome of the conflict.[73]

Given that the waves of pandemic influenza (as determined by pathogen-induced mortality) struck Austrian and German society (and their military forces) before they struck British society, we might expect that influenza debilitated the war effort of the Central Powers more than that of the Allies. Thus, it is variation in mortality and (perhaps even more important) in timing that indicates that Crosby was premature in concluding that all combatants were affected in the same manner. The balance of evidence accumulated herein suggests that the pandemic affected the combatant' militaries, governments, and societies in rather

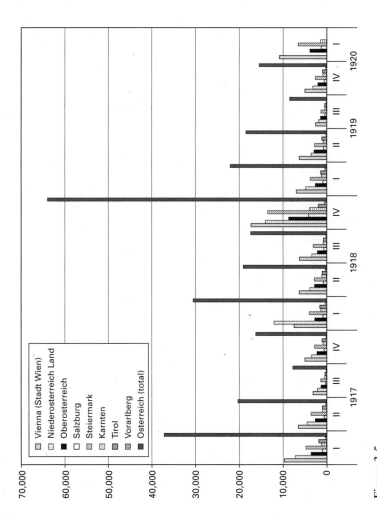

Figure 3.5
Pneumonia mortality, Austria, 1917–1919, by quarter. Source: Same as for figure 3.4.

different ways, and that it may have contributed to the defeat of the Central Powers.

As the data indicate, the contagion eroded the capacity and efficacy of affected militaries, diminishing their optimal functionality. The pandemic's infliction of such debilitation and death on all the protagonists in the war may have effectively brought the conflict to an early end, as military institutions became increasingly sclerotic and ineffective. Moreover, there is some evidence (borne out in the German mortality tables) that the pandemic greatly impeded the German offensive of the spring of 1918, which, if successful, would have resulted in victory for the Central Powers. The second and third waves also diminished German martial power throughout the summer and fall of 1918.

Thus, the epidemic may have prevented a German victory, extended the war, and ultimately assisted in forcing the Central Powers to the table to negotiate peace at Versailles. On October 6 and 7, 1918, at the height of the influenza pandemic in Central Europe, the governments of Germany and Austria sent notices to US president Wilson requesting an armistice and peace negotiations based on Wilson's proposed fourteen points. However, perhaps the most important (and previously unexplored) point is that the visitation of the final lethal viral wave on the immunologically naive population of Austria resulted in widespread death and debilitation and in sclerosis of governance, and ultimately contributed to the collapse of the empire. By articulating this hypothesis I hope to stimulate some debate as to the role of the influenza in the collapse of Austria-Hungary and in the demise of Imperial Germany.

Scapegoating

The history of disease, particularly during its manifestation in European societies, is riddled with fear-induced desires to target minorities as the carriers, instigators, or vectors of disease transmission. It seems a common frailty that humans find it expedient to blame the psychological "other" for visitations of contagion, even pandemic influenza. Despite the fact that the strain may have originated in Kansas (or Austria, for that matter), it was subsequently labeled the Spanish Flu. This designation resulted from the fact that Spain, a neutral party during the conflict, was not actively engaged in the censorship of the reporting of the epidemic at that time. Citizens on the Allied side began to envisage the contagion as some nefarious and demonic weapon conjured by the Germans to poison the people of the Allied countries. For example, one excessively passionate argument went as follows: "Let the curse be called the German plague. . . . Let every child learn to associate what is accursed with the word German not in the spirit of hate but in the spirit of contempt born of the hateful truth which Germany has proved herself to be."[74] While this effect apparently did not result in attacks on demonized minorities (beyond the obvious organized violence directed toward the Central Powers), the central function of contagion-induced stigmatization appears to continue to hold in this case.

Governance

At the domestic level, influenza had a sclerotic effect on governance within severely affected countries, overwhelming the capacity of the state (and often the society) to deal with the debilitation and mortality generated by the contagion. Crosby estimates that the influenza pandemic of 1918–19 generated at least 550,000 excess deaths in the United States (i.e., over and above those deaths that would typically result on an annual basis).[75] As one would expect, one of the first sectors of US society to be overcome was the health sector. Hospitals did not possess the requisite surge capacity to deal with such a huge influx of ill patients. Specifically, hospitals did not possess the necessary beds and supplies, nor did they have adequate reserves of medical personnel (nurses and doctors) on hand to deal with the surge in infected civilians. Moreover, lacking adequate protection, many health providers themselves succumbed to the illness, and thereby became an additional burden on those who remained healthy. The contagion also undercut the timely and effective delivery of other public goods by the state to the people, including essential services such as communications. Crosby notes that "eight hundred and fifty employees of Bell Telephone Company of Pennsylvania stayed home from work on October 7, 1918" and that "on the next day Doctor Krusen of the Department of Health and Charities authorized the company to deny services to any persons making unessential calls, and it presently did so in a thousand cases."[76] This sclerotic effect of the contagion also impacted the police and family services. The pandemic resulted in rampant absenteeism among police officers, firemen, garbage collectors, and social workers to care for children who had lost their parents.[77] Further complicating the situation was the inability to bury the dead promptly and effectively:

The essential service which came closest to collapse in Philadelphia was (morticians). Unless morticians are able to fulfill their duty, two things happen. One, bodies accumulate, creating the possibility of secondary epidemics caused by the various organisms that batten on dead flesh. Two, and more immediately significant, the accumulation of corpses will, more than anything else, sap and even break the morale of a population. When that happens, superstitious horror thrusts common decency aside, all public services collapse, friends and even family members turn away from one another, and the death rate bounds upward.[78]

The discord associated with the pandemic was certainly not relegated to the environs of Philadelphia, but distributed throughout the United States. In the city of San Francisco there were acute shortages of medical personnel, police, communications personnel, educators, and even garbage collectors. "The Sanitary reduction works shut down when only 11 of its normal staff of 56 showed up for work."[79]

While the state's ability to respond was significantly curtailed by the contagion, successful adaptive response came in the form of the mobilization of civil society. It was this galvanic response of non-state organizations, religious, social, economic, and political, that enabled American society to overcome the ravages of the pandemic.[80] Regarding this response by society, it seems reasonable to argue that the civil cohesion generated through the prolonged war effort (notably the Civil Defense Associations) empowered civil society to the extent that it was capable of dealing with the widespread death and disruption generated by the pathogen. It should be noted that different communities responded with varying degrees of effectiveness. San Francisco, for example, was plagued by particularly inept responses, by both civil society and the state. "Despite preliminary planning, organization never caught up with the flu until it had passed its peak. No local Council of National Defense arose to coordinate anti-pandemic forces; no central clearing house to process all calls for assistance . . . was ever created, and San Franciscans ran their doctors ragged checking on cases that needed no professional attention."[81]

The pandemic serves as a prime example of emergent properties, and the Oxford hypothesis supports this line of reasoning. The lethal pandemic influenza of 1918 likely derived its intensity from a combination of the conflict's constituent attributes (and their side effects). Such pernicious factors included the dense troop populations that moved rapidly and continuously around the world (functioning as highly efficient vectors of transmission), coupled with poor nutrition that undermined immune systems, the highly unsanitary conditions of the trenches and military camps, and a novel zoonosis (H1N1 avian influenza). Those permissive conditions, which resulted in rapid viral transmission from host to host, facilitated the evolution of traits of lethality in the virus, resulting in a highly contagious and lethal influenza pandemic. Individually, each one of these constitutive variables may have not generated any significant effect, but when combined in this fashion, led to one of the greatest global public health disasters in recorded history.

Ultimately, the balance of evidence from Germany, Austria, and the United States suggests that the 1918 influenza had various effects on state capacity in affected polities. One obvious effect was that the morbidity and mortality generated by the influenza pandemic generated profound institutional sclerosis. The strongest evidence for this emanates from the extensive problems that became manifest in both the Allied and German military forces during 1918. Other bureaucracies exhibited sclerosis in the United States, particularly those that provided public services such as health care, communication, law enforcement, sanitation, and so forth. Although the preliminary evidence presented here suggests that pandemic influenza did significantly impede the optimal function of state institutions in 1918, further cross-national historical research is required to validate this hypothesis.

The Swine Flu Affair and Its Repercussions

In the wake of the great pandemic of 1918–19, the twentieth century witnessed additional (and relatively minor) pandemics during 1957[82] and 1968.[83] The processes of emergence of pandemic influenza are cyclical and thus, contain a degree of periodicity.[84] However, the Swine flu affair of 1976, which emanated from initial cases of flu-induced mortality in Fort Dix, New Jersey, generated problems in US domestic response to contagion that persist to this day. Despite dire warnings regarding the emergence of a novel strain of highly pathogenic influenza, the 1976 flu failed to generate the high levels of morbidity and mortality that had been predicted. However, profoundly negative repercussions did result from the vaccination program that was authorized by the US government, which rushed though a prototype vaccine without adequate testing before mass dissemination.[85] Owing to the faulty production and insufficient testing of that vaccine, the provision of such vaccinations to the American people resulted in a significant number of people becoming afflicted with Guillain-Barre paralysis.[86] The result was a storm of litigation against the manufacturers, which ultimately resulted in the courts' awarding huge damage settlements to plaintiffs. Ultimately, owing to the litigation, the major US-based developers of vaccines were forced to relocate to Canada and to Europe. This situation persists in the twenty-first century, greatly complicating domestic US ability to respond to a future influenza pandemic. As a result, the US is now almost completely dependent on vaccines produced abroad, and on the honoring of contractual obligations in the face of a global health emergency.

The Future

There is great concern about the geographical spread and the persistence of the H5N1 Avian Influenza that appears to be endogenized within the human ecology of Southeast Asia.[87] The pathogen appears to be a highly lethal[88] zoonosis with the unusual property of being able to jump directly from its natural avian reservoirs into human hosts.[89] The virologists Jeffrey Taubenberger and David Morens argue that, despite our armamentarium of vaccines and antivirals, an emergent influenza pathogen that exhibited lethality of the same magnitude as the 1918 virus would kill more 100 million people today.[90]

In the domain of international commerce, the current strain of avian influenza has already inhibited flows of goods and people to a minor extent. During 2006 the European Union banned imports of poultry and bird products from Bulgaria, including wild birds, eggs, farmed and wild feathered game, and hatching eggs. Further, a regional ban was applied to all imports of poultry meat, eggs, and products from wild fowl. Current EU policies do not provide for compensation to farmers who incur losses as a result of declining public confidence in the safety of poultry.[91] In the European context, the arrival of the virus has already resulted in reduced consumption of poultry, generating hundreds of millions of dollars in losses for that industry.[92] According to the World Health Organization, the disease has already cost 300 million farmers more than $10 billion as a result of its spread through poultry.[93]

Moreover, the next pandemic has implications for the food security of affected countries, as it has already resulted in the culling of millions of birds. Joseph Domenech, chief veterinary officer of the United Nations Food and Agriculture Organization, has cautioned that the spread of the epidemic may undercut nutrition: "If a poultry epidemic should develop beyond the boundaries of Nigeria the effects would be disastrous for the livelihoods and food security of millions of people."[94] This may explain why Nigerian officials were aware of the pathogen within their avian populations for 19 days before informing the public and the international community.[95] Obviously, such deliberate obfuscation and delay can only undercut international attempts at containment.

In 2006, European countries reported the arrival of the H5N1 virus, which has made sporadic appearances in the United Kingdom, France, Germany, Austria, Greece, Italy, Bulgaria, Poland, and Slovenia. Further, the disease is now apparently established in Russia, Ukraine, Romania, Turkey, Bulgaria, Croatia, Egypt, and Azerbaijan (all non-EU countries). EU governments continue to discuss plans to create a pan-European program to vaccinate poultry. In mid February 2006, EU governments announced a program of strict precautionary measures for containment. Specifically, they imposed a general rule that applies and enforces a quarantine and surveillance zone of about 10 kilometers around areas where the virus has been detected.[96]

Containment of the pathogen is likely to be problematic throughout much of Africa, since the slaughter of poultry stocks by government forces is typically not accompanied by reimbursement from the state in this region. As a result, farmers—particularly in Nigeria—have a significant economic disincentive to report unusual avian mortality. This limits surveillance and the execution of containment strategies. Further, many governments in Africa exhibit exceptionally low levels of fiscal capacity, and therefore may be unable to make effective compensation payments. According to former WHO Director Jong Wook Lee, the international community should create a mechanism to cover excess costs associated with such compensation, in order to ensure accurate surveillance and compliance throughout less developed countries.[97]

This situation is complicated by those societies that harbor a legacy of mistrust between civil society and the government, particularly those polities that are in the process of transition from authoritarian rule to nascent democracy. Moreover, the lack of government legitimacy, and education of the population, are also hampering efforts to control the influenza in Nigeria. According to the journalist Dulue Mbachu, "a wall of distrust between the government and most of the population is proving a major obstacle to fighting bird flu in Nigeria. The campaign is also hampered by poor infrastructure, lack of resources, and vast distances. In Nigeria, after decades of misrule by corrupt military and civilian regimes, the 70 percent of the population with little education or income has grown wary of all officialdom."[98]

In the United States, Health and Human Services Secretary Michael Leavitt announced in 2006 that he had authorized the National Institutes of Health and the Centers for Disease Control and Prevention to prepare a second vaccine to counter the H5N1 virus, based on the fact that the prior vaccine was based on samples taken from Thailand in 2004. Health officials now believe that the virus has undergone significant mutation since 2004, and that the form now circulating in Africa and Europe may exhibit significantly greater genetic variance than the prior variant.[99] Although the United States currently possesses a stockpile of 5 million doses of Tamiflu (oseltamivir), in March 2006 it ordered 12.4 million more doses.[100] Unfortunately, recent evidence suggests that certain strains of the virus are highly resistant to oseltamivir, and so the significant expense incurred in stockpiling the compound may not in fact result in the expected positive dividends of protecting the lives of the US public.

Early in 2006, the US Congress authorized $3.8 billion for the purchase of more vaccine and Tamiflu from the Swiss firm Roche and from the British firm GlaxoSmithKline.[101] The central problem emanates from the global competition to procure a rather limited supply of anti-viral prophylaxis, while global production capacity remains inadequate. Compounding the problem, the US federal government has asked the states to create their own individual stockpiles, which may encourage hoarding by wealthier states (such as California and New York). There is currently no federal legal architecture that can compel these states to share their supplies in a cooperative manner to maximize efficiency should a pandemic occur. And there are no substantive international mechanisms to ensure the cooperation of sovereign states.

However, the necessity of developing protocols for international cooperation to combat emerging H5N1 strains has percolated into the upper echelons of the policy-making community, and Paula Dobriansky, former US Undersecretary of State for Global Affairs, has wisely argued for greatly increased international cooperation on the issue.[102] Domestically, the current US strategy is to rely on actions taken abroad to contain the proliferation of the virus, but that is a dubious strategy on several grounds. First, there is enormous variance in the endogenous capacity of foreign states to conduct effective pathogenic surveillance and containment, ranging from the relatively robust capacity of the G-8 countries to the almost non-existent public health infrastructural capacity of states such as Haiti, Ghana, and Cambodia. The situation is exacerbated by perpetually feeble international regimes (including the revised International Health Regulations) and poorly funded international institutions (the WHO). While the WHO was reasonably effective in assisting sovereign states to contain SARS in 2003 (see chapter 5), in recent years the organization has witnessed the re-emergence of poliomyelitis virus in Africa and its spread back to South Asia,[103] an inability to contain the burgeoning HIV/AIDS pandemic, and the continued proliferation of malaria, tuberculosis, and hepatitis around the world.

In the context of such weak international institutions, and with states serving their own material self-interests, we are likely to see less than optimal international cooperation in the face of a highly pathogenic pandemic influenza. The agents of international organizations have admitted as much. Mike Ryan of the WHO recently warned that global capacity for containment of the emerging pandemic is insufficient: "We truly feel that this present threat and any other threat like it is likely to stretch our global systems to the point of collapse."[104] Joseph Domenech, head of the UNFAO's Animal Health Service, complained that the developed world had not done enough to contain the spread of the pathogen throughout the developing world, where countries have insufficient capacity for surveillance and control: "In 2004 we said there will be an international crisis if we don't stop it in Asia, and this is exactly what is happening two years later. We were asking for emergency funds and they never came. We are constantly late."[105]

The primary concern, then, is that a pandemic exhibiting pathogenicity similar to that of the 1918 virus would overwhelm institutions of governance in the G-8 countries, and to an even greater extent in the less developed countries. Arguably, the globalization of tightly coupled economic systems has made us more vulnerable to pathogen-induced disruptions than were our forebears in 1918. Furthermore, such vulnerability is exacerbated by the greatly increased speed of pathogenic transmission, courtesy of modern transportation technologies. Moreover, the SARS epidemic illustrated that the modern media and telecommunications technology may exacerbate economic damage through its rapid diffusion of anxiety, fear, and panic.

Within the United States, the capacity of institutions (both at the state and federal levels) to mitigate the negative externalities associated with an influenza pandemic is very much in doubt. Let us briefly examine the shortcomings at the level of the individual states. According to the dictates of the US Constitution, the individual states possess the legal authority to deal with crises in the domain of public health. However, there is enormous variation among the states in endogenous capacity, including human capital resources (i.e., trained personnel), pathogenic surveillance capacity, fiscal resources, health infrastructure, surge capacity in hospitals, and administrative preparedness for health emergencies. One might simply compare the state of New York, with its vast post-9/11 resources and augmented preparedness, to poorer states, such as North Dakota and New Mexico, which struggle to find the fiscal resources to conduct basic public health surveillance.

At the federal level, the United States' capacity for response is inhibited by a number of factors. First and foremost is the lack of federal powers to deal with a public health emergency, which became quite evident during the Andrew Speaker affair during May and June of 2007. In that particular case, the CDC found itself beholden to the State of Georgia in its attempts to limit the movement of an individual infected with a rare and exceptionally drug-resistant strain of tuberculosis. Certainly, the US Congress could claim jurisdiction over public health emergencies through exercise of the Commerce Clause in order to grant federal bureaucracies such powers.[106] A further problem results from the chronic fragmentation of oversight of health issues among (and within) the various federal bureaucracies, which possess degrees of overlapping jurisdiction in the domains of surveillance, management, and pathogenic containment. For example, the CDC often competes with the NIH within the Department of Health and Human Services over attribution, access to data, and funding. In the face of an avian influenza pandemic, HHS would have to cooperate not only with the states but also with the Departments of Homeland Security, Defense, Agriculture, Interior, Transportation, Commerce, and State. At present there is no cabinet-level official tasked with coordinating a national response, and, as the exceptionally inept federal and state governmental responses to Hurricane Katrina indicated, cooperation between federal bureaucracies and between the federal government and the states cannot be taken for granted. Thus, to optimize the domestic response, a pandemic flu coordinator should be designated at the cabinet level.

In view of the problems evident in US domestic disaster response, the role of civil society remains integral to the provision of effective response in the face of pandemic influenza. In the face of the 1918 contagion, local Civil Defense Associations (i.e., trained civilian volunteers) provided information and assisted beleaguered health-care providers. As Putnam has documented, the gradual erosion of civil society and the consequent erosion of social capital in the United States[107] bode ill for our collective capacity to respond. However, recognizing that civil society may constitute a powerful force for positive intervention, the country should invest in the promotion of preparedness through local civic organizations that can assist the government during such a crisis.

The case of the 1918 pandemic influenza is consonant with a republican reformulation of Realist theory. The pandemic represented a direct threat to the material interests of all countries, political suppression of data often prevented other states from knowing the conditions of affected states, rational decision-making was largely absent, and international cooperation on the issue was non-existent, despite the complex biological interdependence of affected polities.

4

HIV/AIDS, State Capacity, and National Security: Lessons from Zimbabwe[1]

The HIV/AIDS pandemic continues to spread inexorably throughout the developing countries, proliferating from its established base in sub-Saharan Africa to infect millions in India, Eastern Europe, and East Asia. In 2005 the pandemic claimed 2.8 million lives and generated 4.1 million new infections, bringing the number of people currently infected to 38.6 million.[2] Despite the increasing production of anti-viral therapies, access to them remains limited in the developing countries, and resistant strains of HIV have begun to proliferate.

According to UNAIDS' 2006 Report on the Global AIDS Epidemic, the contagion is showing signs of slowing as increases in incidence begin to plateau in certain countries. However, a deeper analysis of UNAIDS' annual data on incidence and prevalence suggests otherwise. Specifically, while there may be selected geographically specific pockets of stabilization (and even amelioration) of HIV, the larger story is one of a pandemic that continues to expand into new geographical domains even as it remains entrenched within its epicenter in sub-Saharan Africa. UNAIDS' interpretation of the data is unusual, as UNAIDS prefers to emphasize the point that the epidemic appears to have slowed its expansion (in terms of prevalence as a percentage of population). However, this is a function of both aggregate population growth and the fact that mortality from HIV/AIDS now equals or exceeds the rate of new infections. Thus, stabilized prevalence does not necessarily equate with an epidemic that has reached an epidemiological equilibrium or "plateau"; it is simply killing more people faster than ever before. (See figure 4.1.)

Globally, the HIV/AIDS pandemic resulted in 4.3 million new infections in 2006, and over 39.5 million people are now HIV positive.[3] Using UNAIDS data on incidence of HIV, I have calculated the rate of

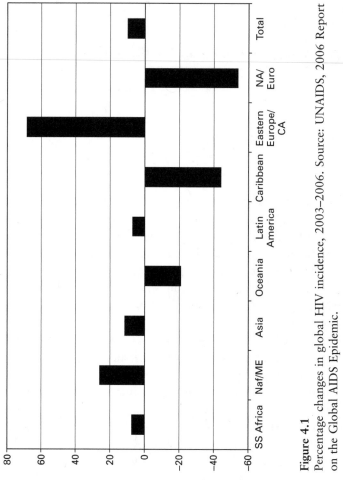

Figure 4.1
Percentage changes in global HIV incidence, 2003–2006. Source: UNAIDS, 2006 Report on the Global AIDS Epidemic.

increase and decrease from 2003–2006, as a percentage, and as defined by geographic region.[4] Enormous variation in incidence has occurred in recent years, the most significant percentage increases occurring in Eastern Europe and Central Asia (68.75), North Africa and the Middle East (25.92), and South and East Asia (11.62). Conversely, the greatest declines were observed in North America and Europe (–53.84), the Caribbean (–44.12), and Oceania (–21.12). Despite the positive nature of such regional declines, certain data are cause for concern. The dramatic gains in incidence across Asia and Eastern Europe indicate that the virus is conquering new territory in the greatest population pools on the planet. This is reflected in the total growth rate, which indicates a substantial 10.25 percent increase globally from 2003 to 2006. Therefore, while the pandemic is certainly declining in certain regions, it continues to accelerate throughout much of the developing world.

Figure 4.2 illustrates regional mortality associated with HIV/AIDS (2003–2006), and the data indicate that the pandemic is far from a state of decline. Calculations indicate that the percentage increase in deaths (2003–2006) was most alarming in Eastern Europe and Central Asia, which saw an increase of 300 percent over that time period. Several other regions also saw increasing death rates (Oceania 73.91, Latin America 58.54, Asia 26.6), while a notable decline was observed in the Caribbean (–47.37). Despite the stabilization of the mortality rate in North America and Europe and the decline in the Caribbean, the aggregate global mortality rate increased over that period by 11.53 percent. This suggests that, in addition to continuing transmission, anti-retroviral therapies are still not reaching many in the developing countries who are infected. Therefore, one must take the ebullient claims of the Joint United Nations Programme on HIV and AIDS (UNAIDS) and the World Health Organization (WHO) with a grain of salt, and conclude that in fact the epidemic shows no distinct indications of slowing transmission on a global scale, nor do we see macro-level reductions in mortality (despite regional pockets of improvement).

Once the greatest success story in Africa, Zimbabwe now totters on the brink of economic and political collapse. The country is now beset by political violence, electoral fraud, foreign wars, and seizures of land from minority whites.[5] Zimbabwe is also beset with a declining GDP, high rates of inflation, persistently high rates of unemployment, increasing poverty, and attenuated drought. Finally, Zimbabwe has one

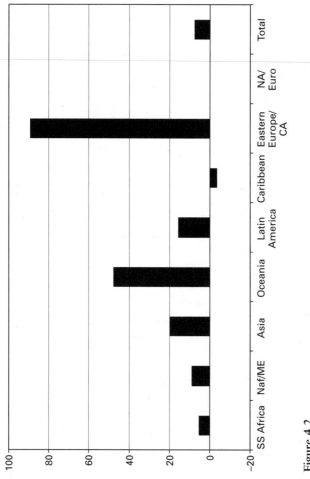

Figure 4.2
Percentage changes in global AIDS mortality, 2003–2006. Source: as for figure 4.1.

of the highest levels of HIV/AIDS seroprevalence in the world, with approximately 20 percent of the population currently infected with the human immunodeficiency virus.[6]

This case study employs process tracing[7] to illustrate the effects of HIV/AIDS on the various domains of economics, governance and security. Within such complex bio-political systems effects may take the form of complex feedback loops and exhibit non-linear properties.[8] Indeed, Margaret and Harold Sprout noted this principal of "connectivity" across domains, stating that "any substantial change in one sector of the milieu is nearly certain to produce significant, often unsettling, sometimes utterly disruptive consequences in other sectors."[9] Moreover, Jervis argues that complex systems exhibit the following properties: "Many crucial effects are delayed and indirect; the relations between two actors (or domains) are often determined by each one's relations with others; interactions are central and cannot be understood by additive operations; many outcomes are unintended; regulation is difficult."[10]

This chapter provides initial empirical evidence of the epidemic's ability to compromise prosperity, political stability and national security in seriously affected regions over the longer term. Given the complex mix of factors working to destabilize Zimbabwe, the HIV/AIDS epidemic should be regarded as a powerful stressor that undermines the prosperity and political stability of that country. In particular I argue that in the context of poor governance (i.e. low levels of political will and state capacity) HIV/AIDS reinforces a vicious spiral within affected societies to threaten the stability of the state.

Literature Review

Historians have long understood the deleterious effects of epidemic disease on the stability of states and societies. The historian William McNeill was explicit on this subject:

The disruptive effect of such an epidemic is likely to be greater than the mere loss of life, severe as that may be. Often survivors are demoralized, and lose all faith in inherited custom and belief which had not prepared them for such a disaster. Population losses within the twenty to forty age bracket are obviously far more damaging to the society at large than comparably numerous destruction of the very young or the very old. Indeed, any community that loses a significant percentage of its young adults in a single epidemic finds it hard to maintain itself materially and spiritually. . . . The structural cohesion of the community is almost certain to collapse.[11]

In recent years infectious disease has gained recognition as a threat to international development and to national security, spurring the development of the nascent field of "health security."[12] Despite the increasingly sophisticated analysis, few studies have assessed the threat as it affects both state and society across domains at the micro and macro levels.[13] Prior analyses have concluded that HIV/AIDS threatens the efficacy of military forces,[14] effective governance,[15] and the macro economy[16] that underpins the preceding variables. The balance of evidence presented herein illustrates that HIV/AIDS constitutes both a direct and an indirect substantive threat to Zimbabwean governance and national security.[17]

Health and State Capacity

I hypothesize that states with relatively low levels of capacity, but governed well, can respond with reasonable efficacy to the epidemic and control its further spread. This has occurred in Thailand, which saw political elites use their power to mobilize civil society in a bid to reduce risky behavior.[18] Both of those countries have seen their seroprevalence levels of HIV infection decline significantly over the past decade. However, countries with middling to low levels of capacity, combined with poor governance, have been ineffective at containing the spread of the contagion, and in mitigating its adverse economic and political effects (e.g., Zimbabwe).

In the context of the HIV/AIDS epidemic this is of utmost importance as it helps to explain differential outcomes in the ability of governments to respond to the epidemic and maintain economic and political stability. For example, Botswana has much better political leadership and higher empirical levels of state capacity than Zimbabwe,[19] despite having a slightly higher HIV seroprevalence rate. It is probable that this combination of effective political leadership and higher endogenous capacity (due to revenues from mineral exports) has moderated the negative effects of the pandemic, whereas Zimbabwe is seeing significant socio-economic destabilization as a result of HIV/AIDS.

This chapter draws on the preliminary finding that there is a strong positive empirical association between population health and state capacity.[20] Population health is measured through indicators of Life Expectancy and Infant Mortality. In an empirical cross-national study of 20 countries, utilizing 40 years of data, Price-Smith demonstrated that public health is a major driver of state capacity. That prior work also revealed the existence of a feedback loop between population health and state capacity, wherein a 15-year lagging of the variables demonstrated that health is a stronger driver of capacity than the obverse. Altogether this suggests that significant declines in population health (regardless of the source of decline) will therefore generate significant declines in downstream state capacity. Given adult seroprevalence rates of 20.1 percent, the HIV/AIDS epidemic has dramatically eroded life expectancy in Zimbabwe and significantly compromised the welfare of the population as a whole.

One might reasonably ask why Zimbabwe seems to be reeling under the epidemic while its neighbor Botswana (possessing a marginally higher adult HIV seroprevalence rate of 24.1 percent) remains generally stable. It seems reasonable to assume that state capacity is an intervening variable between the independent variable of political will on the one hand, and the dependent variable of political stability on the other. Botswana is an interesting case because it is a relatively prosperous rentier state with significant mineral wealth, high per capita income (US$3,100 per annum), and therefore relatively higher levels of state capacity than Zimbabwe. Moreover, Botswana possesses relatively effective political leadership in President Festus Mogae, an Oxford-trained economist who is engaged in efforts to blunt the negative effects of the epidemic on the people of Botswana. The Mogae administration has provided significant leadership in mobilizing communities to reduce endogenous transmission, and has promised that infected persons will receive free antiretroviral therapy to prolong their lifespan and their productivity. Thus, Botswana possesses several critical advantages over Zimbabwe, higher capacity, better political leadership, and greater levels of legitimacy in the eyes of its people.

Health and National Security

The definition of national security has changed over the years to include terrorism, resource scarcity, migration, and now threats to population health. During the first session of the United Nations Security Council of July 17, 2000, the UN adopted Resolution 1308 (2000) and declared the HIV/AIDS pandemic a threat to global security. This represents the first time in history that an issue of public health has been elevated to such status, and it illustrates the recent transformation in thinking about new threats to security in the post-Cold War era.

Robert Ostergard argues, correctly, that security studies have been tainted by an ethnocentric bias that grew particularly acute during the Cold War. Given the bi-polar animosity between the superpowers, Realist theory and praxis emphasized matters of European or North American security, deterrence, polarity, and the relationships between great powers.[21] However, such definitions of security were of little relevance to the peoples of the developing countries, where poverty, disease, famine, and resource scarcity have proved to be perennial threats to "security."

Thus, any agent (e.g., pathogens) that directly threatens to destroy a significant proportion of a state's population base constitutes a significant threat to that state's national security. Insofar as HIV/AIDS is projected to kill more than 30 percent of Zimbabwe's population from 2005 to 2015, it is reasonable to conclude that the epidemic constitutes both a direct and an indirect threat to the national security of Zimbabwe.

While it is now increasingly understood that the AIDS pandemic constitutes a threat to the prosperity, cohesion, and perhaps the security of countries, the process by which the disease destabilizes societies, economies, governance structures, and the national security apparatus remains opaque. Let us delineate the mechanisms by which the contagion undermines prosperity, effective governance, and security. First, the pandemic has dramatically reduced Zimbabwean life expectancy and quality of life, and has produced significant cohorts of orphans, who are extremely vulnerable to radicalization. Second, the destruction of the country's endogenous stock of human capital results in the systematic erosion of the economy through declining productivity, depletion of savings, and a soaring debt. Third, the pandemic is systematically eroding the institutions of governance (such as police and military forces) while depleting aggregate state capacity, thus dramatically narrowing the range of policy options available to policy makers. Fourth, the above factors may combine to exacerbate conflict between elites, classes, and ethnicities, or may foster violence by an increasingly draconian state against its own people in order to maintain control.

Demographic Projections

The HIV/AIDS epidemic has seen significant increases in adult prevalence from an estimated 12 percent of the Zimbabwean population in 1990, peaking at an estimated 33.7 percent in 2001, but declining in recent years to circa 20.1 percent. HIV/AIDS-induced deaths reached their apex in 2001 at an estimated 200,000, and continued at that level through 2003, declining marginally to 180,000 in 2005. More than 800,000 Zimbabweans have died from the disease since 1998. More than 1.7 million Zimbabweans are now infected with HIV, up from 1.6 million in 2003.[22] More than 600,000 have full-blown AIDS, and more than 2,500 die each week as a result of the disease. The epidemic continues to expand throughout the Zimbabwean population, with little evidence of abatement. Within the country the distribution of HIV infection exhibits significant variance, with Masvingo province at 49.4 percent, the midlands at 45.1 percent, and Harare and Bulawayo each at 30 percent.[23]

Zimbabwean life expectancy at birth declined precipitously from 52 years in 1970 to 37 years as of 2006, and it is predicted to fall to 27 years by 2010 according to UNICEF. Indeed, the average Zimbabwean life span decreased by 7.8 years between 1990 and 2006.[24] Infant mortality increased from a rate of 53 deaths per thousand in 1990 to 79 per thousand in 2006, and the mortality of children below the age of 5 increased from 80 per thousand in 1990 to 129 per thousand in 2006, much of which may be attributed to the AIDS epidemic.[25]

As a result of the dramatic winnowing of the adult population, the national population distribution is expected to transform from a pyramidal shape to that of a chimney-type form perched on a large base of children and adolescents. Fourie and Schonteich argue that this demographic shift, and the resultantly large cohort of orphans, has significant negative ramifications for societal stability, as young people are more often involved in criminal activity than older people.[26] Moreover, impoverished and disaffected young people may be convinced to join various radical and destabilizing movements such as militias, paramilitaries, and terrorist organizations.

Orphans

Given that HIV/AIDS generates significant mortality with the 15–45 age range of the population, one might expect the pandemic to generate significant cohorts of orphans who have lost one or both parents to AIDS. UNAIDS estimates the number of Zimbabwean children who have lost one or both parents to AIDS at 1,100,000 as of 2005 (up from 600,000 in 2000).[27] In 2000 the US National Intelligence Council report concluded:

With as much as a third of the children under fifteen in hardest-hit countries expected to comprise a "lost orphaned" generation by 2010 with little hope of educational or employment opportunities, these countries will be at risk of further economic decay, increased crime, and political instability as such young people become radicalized or are exploited by various political groups for their own ends; the pervasive child soldier phenomenon may be one example.[28]

Schonteich has argued that the AIDS epidemic will directly increase the frequency and severity of crime in Zimbabwe in the decades to come, primarily as a function of the inexorably growing population of AIDS orphans: "Growing up without parents, and badly supervised by relatives and welfare organizations, the growing pool of orphans will be at greater than average risk to engage in criminal activity."[29]

The drain of orphaned populations on state coffers will become onerous in the years to come and has the capacity to further strain Zimbabwe's already overtaxed budget. The other portion of the burden will fall on extended families to care for the children, placing additional strains on declining household incomes and savings. Therefore, such a large cohort of orphans threatens to overwhelm already flimsy existing support systems. The majority of these children will grow up impoverished, poorly educated, prone to criminal behavior, and disenchanted with society. As the AIDS epidemic continues to expand, it will destabilize governments throughout the region. Such weakened states may provide fertile breeding grounds for terrorist organizations to move in, set up shop, and recruit from the disaffected, particularly from such enormous orphan populations. This is particularly worrisome given that terrorist organizations are active in eastern Africa and are moving into Southern Africa to set up bases of operations and recruit personnel. Thus, the AIDS orphan problem threatens not only to create governance problems within affected states, but also to contribute to problems of global governance (particularly terrorist activity) in the future.

Economics

Zimbabwe exhibits high levels of income inequality, with approximately 20 percent of the population receiving 60 percent of the income. Roughly 60 percent of the population lives below the poverty line, with the poor spending between 33 percent and 50 percent of their total annual expenditure on food and health care.[30] Zimbabwe is also beset with shortages of foreign exchange, and significant arrears on its foreign debt. What is not often understood is that the HIV/AIDS epidemic has been contributing to the decline of the Zimbabwean economy for some time, exacerbating income inequalities, undermining societal productivity, and generating capital flight out of the country.

Micro-Level Impacts
At the household level, AIDS has a dramatic negative effect on production and earnings, resulting in reduced income, declining productivity, and the reallocation of labor and land to deal with debilitation or death of breadwinners. AIDS-induced debilitation generates a number of negative demand-side and supply-side shocks to households, including the loss of income from infected breadwinners, significant expenditures for medical expenses, and the loss of employment as healthy individuals must care for ill family members. Premature AIDS-induced mortality results in permanent loss of income, large funeral costs, and permanent labor substitution as children are removed from school to generate income for the family. Furthermore, widows may lose their land when their husbands die of AIDS, as male relatives may lay claim to the dead individual's belongings (including their spouses) according to custom. Because most Zimbabwean women lack legal certificates (such as wills or marriage certificates), their rights are not protected.

Moreover, the burden of disease falls unequally on classes, with poorer populations bearing a disproportionate share of the costs relative to their incomes.[31] The indigent may be forced into sexually exploitive situations in order to generate income to make ends meet. The poor will also be most vulnerable to infection given their lower levels of nutrition and lower basal health conditions, and will be unable to afford anti-retroviral therapies that may slow the progression of the disease.

Considerable decline has been witnessed across important sectors ranging from 25 percent of manufacturing capacity since 1998, a loss of 20 percent of mining output volume since 1999, and a decline in earnings from tourism of roughly 50 percent since 1999.[32] This is not to suggest that the AIDS epidemic is responsible for this entire decline in productivity, yet it certainly is a significant factor in limiting the productive possibilities of the Zimbabwean economy. Debilitation and death induce a scarcity of skilled workers and a decline in returns to training. Thus, at the macro level HIV is eroding the endogenous stock of human capital in Zimbabwe. Counter-intuitively, AIDS-induced debilitation and mortality will not dramatically lower the unemployment rate of approximately 45 percent, because as the macro economy contracts this will lower the demand for labor, even as the labor supply diminishes as a result of disease-induced morbidity and mortality. Moreover, there is a pre-existing shortage of skilled labor in the country, and as the epidemic erodes human capital it will only serve to increase the shortage of skilled workers.

Human Capital

Economic development should be regarded as a "generalized process of capital accumulation"[33] wherein capital consists of both physical and human capital and institutions. The epidemic's pernicious influence on the formation and consolidation of human capital within Zimbabwean society is significant. AIDS will take the lives of a significant proportion of the brightest minds of Zimbabwe. This in turn will hamper efforts toward economic development and impede the consolidation of democratic government. It is important to recognize that the HIV/AIDS epidemic simultaneously drains reserves of human capital and prevents its accumulation, combining to weaken a society's institutional capital.

The net outcome of HIV-induced decline in a society's stock of human capital is stagnation of economic development, which over time results in serious economic decline. As government funding is diverted from education to the health-care sector, this dearth of funds will impede the development of human capital, as the young will be increasingly devoid of skills and adequate literacy. McPherson argues that the HIV-induced decline of savings and loss of efficiency is very much like "running Adam Smith in reverse":

As an increasing number of workers become debilitated and drop out of the labor force, many of the advantages of specialization and the division of labor are lost. Moreover, the loss of labor is a direct reduction of the nation's productive capacity.[34]

Thus, the HIV/AIDS epidemic will have a pronounced effect on the accumulation and consolidation of knowledge and skills within the Zimbabwean population while simultaneously depleting the pre-existing stock of human capital through the premature mortality of skilled workers. This long-term process of AIDS-induced human capital erosion will result in significant long-term negative outcomes for Zimbabwean prosperity.

Macroeconomic Impact

As AIDS depletes the national reservoir of human capital and impedes its formation, it will limit the long-term development potential of Zimbabwe. AIDS-induced shortages of skilled workers will result in higher domestic production costs, which will in turn erode international competitiveness. According to estimates by Haacker, the HIV/AIDS epidemic will result in a loss of output per capita (–7.3 percent per annum) resulting from a change in total factor productivity of –1.3 percent.[35] Bonnel estimates that current levels of adult HIV seroprevalence (34 percent) will slow the growth rate of the macro economy, such that disease-induced morbidity and mortality will reduce GDP growth by approximately 1.5 percent per annum.[36] While this may not sound like a significant decline, for the developing countries of southern Africa a 1.5 percent annual decline in GDP growth is an economic catastrophe in the making.

As the rate of population growth declines and the economy contracts, personal incomes, corporate profits, and consumption all will decline. Government revenues are also projected to decline as the tax base stagnates. Simultaneously, the government will attempt to increase expenditure in the health sector, which will result in a deteriorating national fiscal balance. This may result in increased deficit spending in the wake of a contracting endogenous revenue base. Zimbabwe's Gross Domestic Product has declined from US$8.6 billion in 1991 to US$7.2 billion in 2000, which may reflect HIV's increasing drag on national productivity. Similarly, gross domestic investment (as a percentage of GDP) declined precipitously from 20.8 percent in 1981 to 7.8 percent in 2001. Gross domestic savings (as a percentage of GDP) declined over the same period from 14.3 percent to 9.0 percent, while Gross National Savings declined from a high of 12.5 percent in 1991 to 7.4 percent in 2001. This generally reflects the depletion of individual savings by AIDS-induced costs generated by debilitation and premature mortality. Simultaneously, total debt as a percentage of GDP has grown from 39.8 percent in 1991 to 55.8 percent in 2000, although much of this is attributable to excessive borrowing on the part of President Robert Mugabe's regime.[37]

Under the Mugabe regime, Zimbabwe experienced moderate economic success through the 1980s, with GDP growth from 1981 to 1991 averaging a 3.6 percent increase per annum. However, concurrent with the onset of massive infection rates throughout the early and mid 1990s, the annual growth rate of GDP declined to −4.9 percent in 2000, and −8.4 percent in 2001. Moreover, the growth rate of GDP per capita declined from 0.3 percent in 1991 to −7.7 percent in 2000, and to −10.1 percent in 2001. Inflation increased from 32 percent in 1998, to 59.4 percent in 1999, to 108 percent as of late 2001.[38] To offset declining domestic productivity and increased government spending, the Mugabe regime incurred an enormous debt load. The total external debt of Zimbabwe in 2001 was pegged at US$4.45 billion, with debt servicing costs as a percentage of exports running at 69 percent.[39]

In sum, the HIV/AIDS epidemic has already begun to generate serious negative outcomes for the Zimbabwean economy, including declining GDP and GNP in terms of both absolute and per capita measures. It also promises diminishing national and individual savings, declining productivity, and falling rates of foreign investment. The overall picture is one of sustained economic stagnation and accelerating contraction of the economy. Slowing of national economic growth, decline in savings, chronically high levels of unemployment, and declining real per capita GDP will intensify the poverty experienced by the middle and lower classes. The burgeoning epidemic has had a significant negative impact on the economy, and one might reasonably expect HIV-induced economic contraction to intensify in the years to come. Nonetheless, owing to the Mugabe government's increasingly suboptimal economic and political decisions from 1995 to 2008, it is difficult to empirically establish the exact proportion of Zimbabwe's economic decline as a direct result of the contagion. Subsequent studies will require further analysis of this issue.

Foreign Investment
The AIDS epidemic also has had a profound negative effect on the foreign investment climate for Zimbabwe. Prudent foreign investors grow increasingly wary of Zimbabwe's increasingly gloomy economic future, and as a result of the expanding AIDS epidemic they are likely to pull their capital investment out of the Zimbabwean economy.

Alternatively, foreign investors may simply forgo investing in Zimbabwe in favor of countries with lower risk exposures. Significant levels of HIV infection (i.e., seroprevalence exceeding 10 percent) are likely to result in declining levels of foreign investment within seriously affected regions. Notably, the HIV/AIDS epidemic has increased the risk profile for investment in the Southern African region, with investors requiring a premium rate of return exceeding 25 percent throughout Southern Africa.[40] The great uncertainty regarding the ultimate economic effects of the epidemic (attributable to a paucity of information) worsens the investment climate for Zimbabwe, as investors are prudently leery of the unknown. McPherson concurs:

Investors are more likely to wait (defer investment) when they have information indicating that the spread of HIV/AIDS will affect adversely the cost structure of any investment they are contemplating. As the perceived costs of dealing with the spread of HIV/AIDS rises, the rate of investment tends to decline. This has reinforced the decline in the supply of investible resources, already under pressure through falling productivity due to the spread of HIV/AIDS. Thus, while the spread of HIV induces the need for higher rates of investment to help maintain worker productivity, it erodes the means by which such investment can be financed.[41]

As AIDS induces the contraction of the national economy, it will intensify competition between economic and political elites for control over increasingly scarce fiscal resources. This may contribute to substantial governance problems, including increasing the potential for political violence. While detractors of the Mugabe regime might support such political instability as a means of regime change, it is important to understand that any democratic successor regime would also face a similar scenario of continuing economic and political destabilization as the epidemic continues to rage unabated.

National security does not occur in a vacuum, and economic resources are fungible in that they may be readily translated into military power through the acquisition of materiel and the training of forces. Because the AIDS epidemic has the potential to generate significant long-term constraints on the Zimbabwean economy, it will by default place increasing limitations on Zimbabwean military power into the foreseeable future. It is patently impossible to field a modern, well-trained, well-equipped fighting force without a substantial national economic engine to power it. Perversely, this may be a good thing, as the Mugabe regime may be compelled to withdraw its weakening armed forces from foreign theatres of conflict. The AIDS epidemic, with its attendant long-term damage to Zimbabwe's economic base, promises a reduction in the absolute (and perhaps the relative) power of the country over the long term.

Governance

Zimbabwean society today faces immense barriers relating to the practice of good governance. The Mugabe government and its Zimbabwe African Nation Union–Patriotic Front (ZANU-PF) party have systematically implemented strategies to confound democratic governance processes, such as the allowance of basic human rights, the practice of transparency in governmental operations, and free and fair elections.

Suppression of fundamental democratic principles such as freedoms of the press, speech, and public assembly is widespread and is increasing. Recent legislation has further suppressed democratic expression and action. Notably, the Zimbabwean government's Access to Information and Protection of Privacy Act effectively criminalizes free speech, the Public Order and Security Act (POSA) outlaws public meetings, and the Law and Order Maintenance Act (LOMA) prohibits the publication of anything "likely to cause alarm and despondency."[42] This has resulted in the effective censorship of the media and the crushing of dissent within the country.

The Mugabe government employs torture as a tool of political control. It is often used against members of the Movement for Democratic Change (MDC), the main opposition party to the ZANU-PF. Torture, however, is not used only to control opposition party activities. According to Tony Reeler, clinical director for Zimbabwe's Amani Trust, "probably 20 percent of the entire population has had intimate experience with torture."[43]

Governance in Zimbabwe, already exhibiting a significant potential for violence and institutional instability, likely will experience further declines as a result of the AIDS epidemic. The nature of socio-political instability experienced in Zimbabwe today will result in an increasingly demoralized population. This, coupled with rising levels of mortality and morbidity resulting from AIDS, magnifies the sense of hopelessness and despair within the citizenry, and diminishes perceptions of governmental legitimacy. This will create rising individual and collective frustration that will be expressed through increasing acts of lawlessness, personal behavioral recklessness, and callousness toward fellow Zimbabweans. Under these circumstances, one should anticipate growing crime levels, including more aggressive crimes of violence, such as murder and rape.

From 2005 to 2015 Zimbabwe will also lose a substantial portion of its law-enforcement personnel. The Zimbabwe Republic Police serve the needs of Zimbabwe's eight provinces and its two major "provincial" cities, Harare and Bulawayo. Premature loss of personnel will undermine law enforcement's capacity to maintain local peace and tranquility at the community level. The confluence of high and rising unemployment, rampant poverty, rapidly growing cohorts of orphans, severe food and fuel shortages, and an economy in a state of hyperinflation, coupled with the prevalence of HIV, has induced rapidly increasing crime rates.

A comparison of 2001 Interpol crime statistics (the latest available) with those in 1995 exemplifies the degradation that has occurred in Zimbabwe. The population grew 15.5 percent between 1995 and 2001. One might anticipate comparable boosts in crime tied to the growth rate. The incidence of crime grew substantially during this period, as reported murders increased by 68.7 percent during this period, sexual assaults by 26.9 percent, and the incidence of rape by 58.5 percent. Some of this increase might well be tied to the mistaken regional belief that a man can rid himself of HIV by having sexual intercourse with a virgin. The incidence of rape of young girls has soared because of this myth; in some instances, females 5 years old and even younger have been victimized. Other notable increases in criminal activity also occurred during this period include: robbery and violent theft went up 89.8 percent, auto theft 49.1 percent, and aggravated theft 37 percent.[44] These dramatic increases point to a society spiraling into greater lawlessness and social chaos. The growing tendency among the citizenry to shun assistance from law enforcement warrants equal concern. Many victims in Zimbabwe do not report incidents, believing that their calls for aid will be ignored. This is particularly true for those with known affiliations to political, media, or labor factions out of favor with the Mugabe government. The future of effective governance through law enforcement is at risk in Zimbabwe, owing in part to increasing attrition among police personnel. Decline in law enforcement's credibility as a primary source of intervention and assistance to victims of crime explains the growing lack of confidence in this institution.

HIV's Effect on Public Service

The AIDS epidemic affects Zimbabwe's ability to sustain and deliver quality public services for its citizens. Since the early 1990s the Zimbabwean government has been under increased pressure to reform its civil service systems. The World Bank and the International Monetary Fund have linked continued funding to the imposition of structural changes that would reduce Zimbabwe's bloated civil service. Makumbe characterized Zimbabwe's civil service as follows: "weak government capacity to ensure minimal services, highly compressed wages, inability to attract and retain skilled manpower resources, and a large civil service (192,000) absorbing 18 percent of GDP in salary and wages by 1990/91."[45] Recent IMF estimates (October 2000) place Zimbabwe's public service employment at 194,500.[46]

The HIV/AIDS epidemic also has a profound impact on the delivery of public goods and services to the citizenry. Clearly, citizens will pressure the government to spend a greater proportion of national revenue on health provisions. In a country as impoverished as Zimbabwe, there is little elasticity for shifting funds from one revenue source to another.

HIV/AIDS will induce a gradual degradation of the quality of services provided by the bureaucracy. Traditionally, in developing countries like Zimbabwe, educated elites have chosen careers initially in public service. Such employees are often the most highly educated in underdeveloped societies, many having received graduate education from European or American universities. Moreover, these professionals, because of their high incomes, high status in society, and consequently high levels of sexual activity, were earlier victims of HIV than the general population.[47] HIV/AIDS will erode the human capital of Zimbabwe's professional civil service. Costly losses in professional fields (civil engineering, medicine and health care, education, financial administration, developmental planning) are of particular concern.

A significant issue for institutions of governance involves finding adequate replacements to fill the professional lacuna caused by AIDS-induced mortality and morbidity. Certainly, anticipated professional losses ranging as high as 40 percent create great concern about the efficacy of government. Nevertheless, the loss of human capital resulting from HIV/AIDS-related illnesses explains only part of the attrition problems that the Zimbabwean government faces in seeking to maintain institutional viability.

Losses also will result from the voluntary separation of talented public servants who are aware that their HIV status is negative. In part, this exists among individuals who fear that their pensions will have dwindled away by the time they reach their "full-benefits" retirement eligibility status. The political scientist John Daly argues that this occurred in

Swaziland, where highly placed public servants with notable market-ability chose to leave government service early and opted for early retirement and reduced benefits. This occurred because of fears regarding the long-term solvency of their pension plan resulting from the rising numbers of premature medical retirements due to HIV/AIDS.[48]

The crisis identified above attests to the fact that Zimbabwe's government is rapidly witnessing the erosion of its endogenous state capacity. Zimbabwe's level of state capacity determines the scale of adaptive resources that the country could mobilize to mitigate the negative effects of HIV/AIDS. In this instance, the Zimbabwean government has clearly failed the task. Therefore, its society faces a vicious spiral in the form of a positive feedback loop. As the AIDS epidemic progressively takes its toll, Zimbabwe's state capacity declines, and as Zimbabwe's state capacity declines its ability to institute creative AIDS intervention strategies correspondingly diminishes.

The government's ability to deal effectively with the AIDS epidemic is also hampered by its declining financial capacity. Realistically, under the best of financial conditions, Zimbabwe would have a difficult time developing adaptive strategies to curtail effectively its HIV/AIDS epidemic. Burdensome debt obligations to international financiers, including the World Bank and the International Monetary Fund, stunt the implementation of effective health interventions and progressive educational awareness initiatives. These debts divert monies away from health programs toward repayment schemes. At the beginning of 2000, for example, Zimbabwe expended 25 percent of its export earnings to service its debt, even as an estimated 28 percent of its population was infected with HIV/AIDS.[49] The combination of declining fiscal health and state capacity render successful endogenous adaptive HIV/AIDS strategies by the Zimbabwean government unlikely in the near future. This decline in capacity, coupled with a government and an economy on the verge of collapse, suggests that exogenous assistance from developed countries, UN agencies, and major private sector donors will be necessary to avert further degradation of Zimbabwe's socioeconomic and political structures.

As HIV erodes state capacity, it undermines the state's ability to provide public goods to the population (e.g., health care, education, law enforcement), which in turn accelerates HIV proliferation in a negative spiral. Therefore, purely endogenous strategies to build capacity and curb the spread of the epidemic are unlikely to be successful, and capacity will have to be imported from exogenous sources (such as foreign aid). Thus, the desire for purely "African solutions" to the HIV epidemic, while understandable, have been of limited utility, as advocates fail to acknowledge the epidemics inexorable and negative effect on endogenous state capacity. Furthermore, with many societies in sub-Saharan Africa now reeling under the strain of HIV/AIDS, the cumulative effect will be to erode the capacity of the region as a whole. Affected states will find it increasingly difficult to come to each other's aid.

In a climate of increasing lawlessness, a stagnant or contracting economy, increasing institutional fragility, and declining tax revenues, the capacity of the state will be, at a minimum, strained. There are increasing demands on the state from all sectors to deal effectively with the epidemic, even as the epidemic inexorably erodes the state's capacity to respond effectively. Simultaneously, as the population becomes increasingly infected, morbidity and mortality will grow, poverty will deepen as people deplete their savings, and crime will increase. All of this will result in increased feelings of relative deprivation and injustice on the part of the people, who increasingly perceive the government as illegitimate. It is precisely this combination—a weakening state and increasing real and/or perceived deprivation—that increases the probability of political violence within that society, and between society and the state.[50]

History has shown that outbreaks of epidemic disease often result in the curtailing of civil liberties.[51] Thus, HIV/AIDS may induce a shift from democratic to more authoritarian modes of government, particularly in unstable nascent democracies. Indeed, in a climate of disease-induced disorder, scarce resources, and declining government legitimacy, the state may increasingly resort to violence against competing factions within its own population in an attempt to maintain order.[52] Epidemic disease has generated stigmatization and conflict between rival ethnicities over the centuries, typically with the scapegoating of minority populations, such as the whites in Zimbabwe. While there is little evidence that the Shona and the Ndebele consider white populations to be the cause (or the principal carriers) of the disease, affluent white populations have been targeted for political violence as the majority sinks deeper into poverty and chaos. As the epidemic continues to intensify and generate increasing deprivation for the majority, there is every reason to believe that violence against white minority populations will increase, particularly if the Mugabe regime continues to employ such tactics as a means to distract the people from their many grievances. Notably, in December 2000, Mugabe publicly stated to a ZANU-PF Congress: "Our party must continue to strike fear in the heart of the white man, our real enemy."[53]

Increasing disease-induced deprivation combines with a weakening state to generate an increasing probability of violence within the society, either among ethnic groups, among classes, or among political elites. It may also foster the deliberate use of violence by the state against its own citizens in an attempt to retain control. This phenomenon is widely observed throughout Zimbabwe. As the state becomes increasingly unable to satisfy the demands of the people, it is seen as increasingly illegitimate. It is apparent that the Mugabe government is resorting to violence against the population. Thus, as the epidemic intensifies, one would expect an intensification of authoritarian rule as the government becomes ever more desperate to hold onto power.

National Security

The "securitization" of HIV/AIDS has become an issue of significant debate between the paradigms of "national security"[54] and "human security."[55] Orthodox conceptualizations of national security are overly militaristic and myopic, ignoring a plethora of issues (such as environmental change, disease, and migration issues) that threaten states in the modern era. Conversely, while human security arguments may be intuitively appealing, Roland Paris has argued that they present significant conceptual and analytical hurdles.[56]

In relative terms, the absolute mortality that AIDS has induced within the Zimbabwean population vastly exceeds deaths resulting from any armed conflict in the recorded history of that country, and it is increasingly common to hear Zimbabweans refer to the epidemic as a "holocaust." Moreover, the epidemic's contribution to demographic contraction, economic destabilization, and sclerosis in governance directly threatens the material interests of the state, and of Zimbabwean society. Thus, HIV/AIDS has a direct negative effect on Zimbabwean security.

In many countries, military and law-enforcement forces serve as control mechanisms to ensure and sustain the peace within society. In Zimbabwe, however, these units also function as instruments of terror. President Mugabe and the ZANU-PF party use them to prop up and fortify an illegitimate government, which faces claims that it stole the national presidential election in March 2002 through corruption, vote rigging, and voter intimidation.[57] Moreover, the Mugabe regime apparently continues such practices as it subverted the democratic process in the March 2008 general elections and kept the MDC from attaining power.

The nascent literature on health security views AIDS-induced destabilization as contributing to intra-state and inter-state conflict. Elbe and Ostergard have argued that AIDS-induced mortality and morbidity jeopardize the efficacy of military institutions and may thereby promote conflict between states.[58] Elbe argues that AIDS is eroding the functional efficacy of African military institutions along four dimensions:

[AIDS generates] the need for additional resources for the recruitment and training of soldiers to replace those who have fallen ill, have died, or are expected to die. . . . Additional resources are also required to provide health care for soldiers who are sick or dying. Second, the spread of HIV/AIDS is affecting important staffing decisions. High HIV prevalence rates lead to (1) a decrease in the available conscription pool from which to draw new recruits (2) deaths among officers higher up the chain of command, and (3) a loss of highly specialized and technically trained staff who cannot be easily or quickly replaced. Third . . . it can result in increased absenteeism and reduced morale. Fourth, HIV/AIDS is generating new political and legal challenges for civil-military relations. . . .[59]

A 2001 estimate by South Africa's Institute for Security Studies places the respective sizes of the Zimbabwe National Army (ZNA) and the Air Force of Zimbabwe (AFZ) at 35,000 and 4,000.[60] Historically, military and paramilitary organizations have also served as primary vectors for the spread of sexually transmitted pathogens, including HIV. In 2001, according to estimates by the political scientist Lindy Heinecken, Zimbabwe's armed forces had an aggregate seroprevalence rate of 55 percent.[61] Extensive planning will be needed now to replace the losses of more than 1,000 professionally trained personnel per year just to maintain minimal levels of professional competency. In Zimbabwe, HIV-related military attrition will create a loss of continuity at the command level and in the ranks as experienced higher-ranking officers are forced into early medical retirement. The military analyst Rodger Yeager of the Civil-Military Alliance to Combat HIV and AIDS notes that military staff attrition also results in "increased recruitment and training costs for replacements, and a general reduction in preparedness, internal stability, and external security. In this sense, HIV/AIDS can easily serve as a domestic and regional destabilizer and a potential war-starter."[62] Thus, Mugabe's military strength, which serves as an instrument of control over legitimate democratic processes, will slowly and almost invisibly erode over the next decade. Losses of more seasoned and experienced military staff through HIV- and AIDS-related attrition will induce institutional fragility in the apparatus of coercion.

In 1998, Zimbabwe dispatched military personnel and arms to fortify the Democratic Republic of the Congo (DRC) in support of the regime of Laurent Kabila.[63] By 2001, 8,000 members of the Zimbabwe military were deployed to the DRC.[64] Deployment of Zimbabwean military personnel further compounds the transmission of HIV, as separation from one's family often results in increased sexual contact with prostitutes and other high-risk partners. The fact that other sexually transmitted diseases often go unchecked within this group, especially during active military conflicts, exacerbates the problem. Estimates have placed HIV seropositivity levels of the Zimbabwe servicemen returning from the DRC as high as 80 percent.

Zimbabwe's Air Force also will degrade substantially without a plan that overcomes likely human capital losses caused by HIV and AIDS. Compulsory HIV screening, mandated for US military personnel, is not utilized in Zimbabwe's Army, but it is selectively utilized in its Air Force. For example, Air Force aircrew and medical officers receive regular testing. HIV-positive pilots and medical officers are subject to grounding, reassignment, and eventual discharge.

Beyond the loss of gifted professionals and seasoned military leaders, the AIDS-induced erosion of human capital creates broader problems for Air Force and Army operations. It creates major gaps for sustaining crucial operational aspects of these services. For example, morbidity- and mortality-induced losses of technical talent (e.g., airplane mechanics, computer and information specialists, accountants, procurement officers) weaken the service and the mission of these organizations. According to John Daly, AIDS-induced losses in the Zimbabwe Air Force (AFZ) from 2004 to 2014 will range from 1,300 to 2,600.[65]

In the case of Zimbabwe, the progression of AIDS will weaken the military and its capacity to sustain national security. Although AIDS-induced mortality has certainly weakened the power of the Zimbabwean state relative to its regional rivals, there is no empirical evidence that the rising levels of contagion will precipitate war between sovereign states. This results from the fact that other proximate states are also confronting the operational difficulties associated with the contagion, such that external military adventures are becoming prohibitively costly for all affected states in the region. Further, those states that exhibit lower rates of infection, and therefore increasing relative power, will be reluctant to conduct martial campaigns in affected territories, fearing the infection of their soldiers. Moreover, the subsequent demobilization may intensify transmission within the aggressor state. This is not to say, however, that the rising levels of disease will equate with pacific relations within the state.

Violent Intra-State Conflict

HIV/AIDS will have a significant long-term negative effect on the prosperity and the quality of life of the majority of the Zimbabwean people, generating increasing levels of relative deprivation throughout the population. Relative deprivation will increase for the lower and middle classes, which bear a relatively greater cost of AIDS-induced morbidity and mortality. All Zimbabweans will experience absolute deprivation as the economy stagnates and begins to contract. Increasing deprivation generates increasing frustration and aggression in both individuals and collectivities, increasing the probability of social violence and political chaos.[66] However, if deprivation were the sole sufficient and necessary condition to generate political violence, the majority of states in the world would be perpetually consumed within the fires of internal rebellion. This is certainly not the case. Collective violence against the state tends to occur when stressors (such as the HIV/AIDS epidemic) create both the incentive and the opportunity for citizens to engage in violent collective action against the status quo. Thus, the strength or weakness of the state apparatus is a major factor in whether men decide to rebel against their political masters. When increasing deprivation is combined with declines in state capacity and legitimacy, these factors act together to increase the probability of collective violence against the state, or societal factions affiliated with the state.

The AIDS epidemic will generate increased competition between interest groups for increasingly scarce economic resources, particularly as federal funding is diverted to health care and away from other sectors such as law enforcement, education, and the military. The epidemic has certainly placed rapidly increasing demands on the Zimbabwean government to provide additional services to its population, even as the government's capacity to provide such additional services is simultaneously reduced by the expanding AIDS epidemic. Furthermore, the federal government may have to significantly increase taxation of the population to restore depleted government coffers. This resulting reduction of services and increasing taxation in a climate of increasing deprivation will further erode the government's legitimacy. Thus, the AIDS epidemic will simultaneously increase absolute and relative deprivation, increase perceptions of government ineptitude and illegitimacy, and erode state capacity, increasing the probability of internal collective political violence against the state, or intensify violence by the predatory state against its own population. Thus, the HIV/AIDS epidemic may not only kill and impoverish a significant proportion of the Zimbabwean people; it may also contribute to macro-level political and social destabilization that will jeopardize the stability and security of the country.

Effects on Regional Stability

With increasing HIV/AIDS infection throughout sub-Saharan Africa, the pandemic threatens to destabilize many countries in the region, including Botswana, South Africa, Zambia, Angola, Malawi, Namibia, and Mozambique. The epidemic is also burgeoning in Nigeria, Kenya, Tanzania, Swaziland, and Lesotho. As the pandemic crests in the region, it increases the potential for the economic and political destabilization of the Southern Cone of Africa. This bodes ill for the spread and consolidation of democracy and provides fertile ground for the spread and consolidation of radical and/or terrorist operations.

One important element in the discussion of infectious disease's impact on national security is its possible effect on the relative power of states, particularly within a regional context. Certainly the HIV/AIDS epidemic will reduce Zimbabwe's absolute power over the long term, with its profound and negative effects on the country's military and its economy. With respect to Zimbabwe's relative power (that is, its power relative to other states), the equation will be increasingly complex as a function of varying HIV infection rates throughout sub-Saharan Africa. This means that the pandemic will have a greater negative effect on the relative power of Zimbabwe than on neighboring states such as South Africa and Mozambique, which have lower HIV/AIDS prevalence rates. Zimbabwe's power relative to Botswana and Zambia (which have similar prevalence rates) will remain essentially unaltered by the AIDS epidemic, even as the absolute power of these countries is diminished by the contagion. The point here is that high levels of lethal epidemic disease can erode a state's absolute power and, more importantly, erode a state's power relative to its rivals.[67] Though it is unlikely that contagion-induced shifts in relative power will generate interstate war, it is important to note that the epidemic has the long-term potential to alter regional balances of power and the ability to project power. (This finding will become increasingly important as the pandemic intensifies in other states, including India, Russia, Ukraine, and China.)

The AIDS-induced decline of effective governance throughout the Southern Cone will require an increasingly effective military to guarantee the integrity of regional borders. Unfortunately, as was shown above, HIV's negative effect on the military promises increasing "institutional fragility" for that institution and diminishing levels of tax revenue to direct toward military funding as a result of the declining economy. Thus, while the required demand for military power and efficacy is growing, the supply of military power and efficacy is rapidly declining as a result of the epidemic's effects on military personnel. As a result, Zimbabwe should be increasingly concerned that the regional epidemic promises increasing insecurity for the country as a result of both internal and external destabilization. The greatest immediate risk is increasing instability throughout border regions as a result of crime, smuggling, and refugee movements.

A frequently asked question is "At what threshold might HIV seroprevalence (as a percentage of population) cause a society to experience the collapse of effective governance?" The answer remains elusive, as it depends on whether the population has access to effective anti-retroviral therapies, whether the government will provide such therapies to infected populations in a comprehensive and non-partisan manner, and to what extent the economy, governmental institutions, and legitimacy have been damaged by the epidemic. It may also depend on regime type, as nascent democracies and authoritarian regimes will likely exhibit different vulnerabilities to disease-induced economic and political destabilization. Established democracies would seem to be more resistant to such disease-induced stresses. It is necessary to understand the effects of HIV from the perspective of an "attrition process" entailing slow and inexorable destruction of a country's economy, institutions, and social mores. The pandemic is an attenuated process, not a temporally constrained event.

The global HIV/AIDS pandemic would also seem to exhibit emergent properties as it involved the zoonotic transmission of a virus (likely from primate populations) into the human ecology, was transmitted globally via rapid air transportation, established local transmission via sexual conduct and drug use, and exploded within dense urban population pools. It was the combination of these pivotal factors that led to the emergence of this pandemic.

This chapter demonstrates the means by which pathogenic infection acts across domains (demographic, economic, and governmental institutions) to compromise governance and ultimately the national security of seriously affected societies. It also provides preliminary evidence that HIV/AIDS-induced declines in population health are generating a significant decline in State Capacity, and increase in political turbulence within Zimbabwe.[68] These findings permit the formulation of a set of axioms regarding the effects of HIV/AIDS on governance[69]:

• Demographic collapse will generate vast cohorts of orphans, who may then generate crime and/or be radicalized.
• The burden of illness falls disproportionately on the poor, exacerbating inequities between classes.
• Economic contraction generated by the HIV/AIDS contagion will lead to competition over scarce resources, fostering competition between elites, classes, and possibly ethnicities.
• Disease and conditions generated by it foment scapegoating and persecution of ethnic minorities.
• AIDS-induced mortality erodes the base of endogenous human capital, constraining future economic productivity and generating institutional fragility throughout existing structures of governance.
• As the contagion withers institutional capacity and erodes the economy, it may alter the relative power of affected states vs. non-affected states, although this does not generate inter-state warfare.
• The pernicious effects of AIDS radiate across domains to undermine the cohesion of both state and society, and the Zimbabwean government has resorted to the draconian use of lethal force against its own people. This has in turn, inspired further resistance against a state that is widely viewed as illegitimate. This illustrates the persistence of contagionist thought.

In sum, the HIV/AIDS pandemic represents a significant threat to the population of seriously affected societies, particularly those with low levels of state capacity and poor leadership. Thus, the pandemic repre-sents both a direct and indirect threat to the material interests, political stability, and thus the national security of affected states. The persistent lack of effective cooperation among states to check the spread of the pandemic, the political suppression of data, and the opposition by many affected states to external assistance all support a republican theoretical model.

5

Mad Cows and Englishmen: BSE and the Politics of Discord

Fear and economic dislocation gripped British and then other European populations throughout the latter half of the 1990s as a result of the emergence of a novel epizootic, generated by infectious prions, that generated "scrapie" in sheep, Mad Cow Disease in bovines, and the horrific Variant Creutzfeld-Jacob Disease in humans. Bovine Spongiform Encephalopathy ("Mad Cow Disease") is a uniformly lethal disease of cattle that is generated by prions (rogue proteins that infect normal proteins and cause them to shift their structure or alignment to a malign form). The malignant protein then causes significant damage to the cellular structures of the brain of the infected host. Over time, this damage manifests in a progressive loss of motor control, and ultimately in death. Although classified as pathogenic, prions are not understood as infectious" in the normal sense of the term as it is applied to other infectious diseases discussed herein. Nonetheless, prions are transmissible, and their vectors of transmission remain opaque.

BSE would seem to have resulted from the suspect practice of feeding cattle meat-and-bone meal that contained prion-laden offal from infected sheep.[1] Since the mid 1980s, it has become evident that prions appear to be capable of jumping the species barrier from sheep to cattle through processes of zoonosis. Prions have sporadically colonized small groups within the human ecology, often via the global human food supply. Consumption of prion-tainted meats may result in infection of the human host and in subsequent manifestation of prion-induced illness, which is characterized as Variant Creutzfeld-Jacob Disease (VCJD). Eventually, human victims uniformly fall prey to catastrophic neurological damage, which manifests in a decline of mental capacity and motor function and ultimately leads to the rather gruesome death of the host.

As of December 8, 2005, approximately 187,000 cases of BSE had been reported in cattle, spanning 26 countries, with 97.86 percent of those cases occurring in Britain. As of early 2006, approximately 160 human individuals had been diagnosed with VCJD, more than 90 percent of them in Britain.[2]

On Fear and Risk

Historically, fear has been the handmaiden of contagion, amplifying the initial effects of the empirical morbidity and mortality generated by the pathogenic agents in question. Human populations in the past exhibited fear in the face of the uncertainty generated by novel agents of contagion, and this process remains very much in effect in the modern era, particularly when societies are presented with a lethal, incurable, and poorly understood pathogen such as prions. The level of fear experienced on a collective or societal level seems to be a direct function of the levels of uncertainty associated with the emergence of a new disease, inhibiting effective calculations of risk.[3]

Thus, inaccuracies in the perception (and more often misperception) of risk becomes central as an explanatory variable, particularly in the case of Bovine Spongiform Encephalopathy (BSE). BSE is indeed a classic case of the perils of trans-boundary risk management, with high levels of uncertainty, which have persisted over time, and with significant perceptions of risk, both to national economies and to human health. Such perceptions of risk, and the attendant fear, are accentuated by a lack of vaccines to prevent transmission. Moreover, there are no cures for transmissible spongiform encephalopathies as a class of illnesses, nor are there any tests (ante-mortem) to determine whether an animal (or a human) has the condition.

As Richard Posner notes, individuals tend to overweight risks associated with phenomena (such as pathogen-induced mortality) that are considered "dreadful" and "unknown."[4] Cass Sunstein explains that the inaccurate assessment of such risk often stems from "probability neglect."[5] Cognitive factors may also inhibit the human capacity to assess risks associated with novel pathogens. Posner argues that humans exhibit "imagination cost."[6] Prions, and the disease induced by such novel pathogens, certainly are novel and dreadful, and certainly would qualify.

BSE in the European Union

Britain began its arduous trials with BSE (and VCJD) in the mid 1980s, although there were sporadic reports that BSE may have existed in British cattle stocks for some time before that. The first documented case of BSE was apparently diagnosed in Sussex County in 1984.[7] From that date the number of cases confirmed by the British government continued to proliferate until they exceeded 15,000 by April 1990. At that point the crisis was severe enough that the European Commission immediately imposed a ban on exports of live cattle from Britain, and mandatory registration of all BSE cases. Dissembling and obfuscation became the stock in trade for the British government during this period, as the British Minister of Health was quoted in December of 1995 as having said "there is no conceivable risk of BSE being transmitted from cows to people."[8] However, the lie was revealed in March 1996, as the Ministry of Health thereupon informed Parliament that a spate of new clinical diagnoses of VCJD in Britons probably was related to exposure to BSE.

As with other manifestations of infectious disease, the affective component, in this case extreme levels of fear and anxiety, came to the forefront of British society. Uncertainty over whether one was infected, inflamed by rampant media sensationalism, undermined rationality among the public. According to the historian John Fisher, in 1996 "the public sense of unease which had been simmering—and flaring regularly—now erupted in hysteria. Beef sales fell precipitously, and not only in Britain. Cattle production and marketing were thrown into chaos; the already delicate relationship between Britain and its partners in the European Union was brought under further strain when a total ban on the export of British cattle and beef was instituted."[9] The historian John Fisher contends that the British Ministry of Agriculture, Fisheries and Food (MAFF) was completely ineffective in the initial phases of the crisis:

MAFF failed to gain or enforce compliance with its regulations in virtually every area of concern. With compensation payments often inadequate, notification of BSE has been haphazard and the export certification system has been rife with evasion. An audit in 1994 could not account for half of the specified bovine offal (SBO) from slaughtered cattle. The amounts involved were massive and the Assistant Chief Veterinary Officer conceded that most would have gone into animal feed. Claims for the perfect safety of British beef were nonsense. The gap between regulation and actual practice was glaring.[10]

After the revelation of the true extent and depth of the BSE problem in British cattle stocks in March, British Meat and Livestock Commission statistics indicate, the price of retail beef declined by 11 percent in 1996, and the consumption of beef products declined by 24 percent, demand having shifted to other foodstuffs.[11]

The crisis also had significant effects on the British government, as the people lost trust in their elected officials and in the "scientific experts" that had reassured them that BSE could not jump the species barrier and therefore posed no threat to human health. Collectively this contributed to a crisis of legitimacy. The government was seen as abrogating its duty to protect the commonweal, and the scientific community was derided as either ignorant, deliberately callous, or the pawn of agribusiness interests. O'Neill concurs and argues that the crisis led to a "loss of consumer confidence . . . and potentially more seriously, a loss of public trust in government regulators to maintain food safety. This was seen to maximum effect in the response of the British public to the government's delayed announcement of the transmission of BSE to humans."[12] The BSE crisis therefore contributed to a dramatic decline in the perceptions of the legitimacy of the state by the affected British population. Fisher concurs, arguing that "the Conservative government, and especially MAFF . . . employed *suppresio veri* and *suggestio falsi* in order to downplay the scale of the BSE epizootic and the risk of transmission to humans in order to protect the interests of the cattle producers. Governments and their agencies have an evident and natural interest in minimizing public alarm in conditions of uncertainty, but this does not necessarily correspond to deliberate misinformation."[13] Such behavior on the part of the British state exacerbated the historical tensions between state and society in the face of epidemic disease. Ultimately, the actions of the British state reinforced the perception that the state will adopt Machiavellian and contagionist tactics in order to maintain control and protect the interests of vested and powerful domestic elites. "As knowledge of regulatory inadequacies has grown," Fisher writes, "it has reinforced skepticism and suspicion of government and government agencies to the point where they have come to be considered the cause of the problem rather than merely an exacerbating factor."[14]

The BSE contagion destabilized economies and undermined the legitimacy of governments, but in the Schumpeterian sense of "creative destruction" it also provided a window for institutional change, particularly at the domestic level of governance. In the United Kingdom, the

BSE crisis significantly undermined the trust of the people in government institutions (particularly MAFF), and shattered the public's perceptions of the scientific community as both knowledgeable and trustworthy. Therefore, epistemic communities, at least in the case of animal husbandry and public health, were seen as either corrupt or incompetent. As a result, the BSE crisis set the stage for the dissolution of MAFF, which proved itself incompetent again in the foot-and-mouth disease epidemic of 2001. At that point in time, the organization had proved itself so persistently incompetent, and beholden to various interests, that it was dissolved and its functions transferred to the nascent Department for Environment, Food, and Rural Affairs in 2001.

On March 27, 1996, the European Union imposed a complete ban on beef products from Britain, whereupon it conducted surveillance of British efforts in order to ensure that London was truly dealing with the problem in the most effective and timely manner. Despite the increased surveillance, from 1996 onward BSE began to spread from its base in Britain throughout the other countries of the European Union, resulting in a 30 percent collapse in the market price of beef in 1997 as the problem became evident throughout Europe. As the spread of BSE was documented throughout the European Union, exports from EU members to non-EU countries such as Russia were summarily banned by the latter. The decline in beef prices was particularly acute in Germany, where prices tumbled by circa 50 percent in 1997 as citizens reacted against the false claims of their government, which had gone to some lengths to assure the people that the food supply was untainted.[15] The proliferation of BSE throughout Europe generated considerable acrimony between various EU countries throughout the latter half of the 1990s, both bilaterally and multi-laterally. Of particular note was the discord generated between Britain and France. French Agriculture Minister Jean Glavany took an active part in the polemics, stating: "Our English friends exported this evil. . . . They should be morally condemned for this. They spread the animal feed through export which caused it to cross borders even while banning these feeds domestically."[16] In 1998, members of the British Parliament attacked other EU countries (France in particular) for maintaining the ban on UK exports, accusing them of putting narrow political and economic self-interest ahead of science. "I am satisfied," said the British Agriculture Minister at the time, Jack Cunningham, "that there are no grounds for continuing with the totality of the ban. The decision should be taken on a scientific basis."[17] Negative perceptions of

British actions damaged relations with other EU countries, such as the Netherlands. Laurens Jan Brinkhorst, Minister of Agriculture for the Netherlands, commented on the massive cull of livestock in Britain and the incineration of the bodies in vast pyres: "The mass slaughter of healthy animals led to public outrage and I take this very seriously."[18] Protests by domestic factions or stakeholders added additional complexity to the situation, acting in collective fashion to reinforce negative images of the "other," whether that other was a foreign country, or indeed their own de-legitimized state.[19]

In late October of 1999, French farmers initiated an illegal blockade of French ports and set up a cordon to search incoming shipments of goods for British agricultural exports. Such actions were rationalized by the participants as justifiable retaliation for an earlier boycott of French goods by consumers in the United Kingdom.[20] Fear and anxiety swept across France during the fall of 2000. BSE had begun to proliferate among French cattle stocks, resulting in the collapse of beef sales and prices. Domestically, this generated considerable acrimony within France between consumers and producers, and within the various factions of the French government. President Jacques Chirac appeared on French television to discuss the crisis on November 19, 2000. He demanded an immediate ban on all meat and bone meal (MBM) feedstocks, and called for rigorous and comprehensive testing of all domestic cattle. This generated a hail of criticism from Prime Minister Lionel Jospin, who perceived Chirac's moves as an attempt to usurp his position. Jospin railed against Chirac for exacerbating the "collective psychosis" gripping the country in order to make political gains: "It is not the role of leaders to frighten public opinion."[21] By late 2000 it was apparent that the French government was falling victim to the same crisis of legitimacy that had haunted the British government for its failure to deal with BSE.

The European Union concluded in late 1998 that proper safeguards had finally been enacted by the United Kingdom, and subsequently the European Union recommended to its member states that the ban on British cattle and beef products be lifted as of August 1, 1999. However, France chose to ignore this EU ruling, and permitted UK beef to cross its territory but not to enter the French food supply. The European Commission then initiated legal action against France for failure to comply with its obligations as a member state.[22] Within France the crisis also pitted domestic interest groups against one another. "The BSE crisis," Patrick Messerlin noted, "has dealt a fatal blow to the longstanding love affair between French consumers and farmers. In December 2000, farmers blocking roads in northern France were accused of being 'poisoners' on French radio waves—an accusation reminiscent of the revolutionary 1780s."[23]

According to Michel Setbon et al., the BSE crisis generated an enormous sociopolitical and economic crisis in France after the discovery of BSE contamination of endogenous French stocks.[24] Its profound impact resulted from the combination of a novel pathogen (prions), which generated high levels of uncertainty (particularly regarding the extent of infection of the people), combined with anticipated high levels of lethality. As in Britain, the crisis generated enormous levels of affect (emotion) that ranged from to fear, to anxiety, to anger.[25] These powerful affective currents in French society combined with the discovery of a BSE-positive cow in a French slaughterhouse in November 2000 to cause the price of beef in France to plunge by 20–30 percent.[26] Echoing the British case, the crisis also served to undercut society's perceptions of the trustworthiness and legitimacy of the state. Setbon et al. argue that "in spite of numerous official informative campaigns and preventive measures, suspicion (of the food supply) was durably established."[27] Indeed, they argue that society's perceptions of the state in the aftermath of the crisis "seems to be structured by a permanent feeling of social distrust. . . . This is probably because people judge the magnitude of the human epidemic unchanged by (the state's) decisions and consider that public authorities are still to be blamed."[28] Messerlin concurs that the BSE crisis also undercut perceptions of legitimacy of the French government:

... the BSE crisis again underlines the low accountability of French governments—and of the European Commission. . . . Since the late 1980s, all French agriculture Ministers have fought, delayed and limited all necessary measures for protecting human health. French governments have also failed to take necessary anti-BSE measures even several years after Britain did. France (banned MBMs) in July 1990, but only for bovines—a disastrous limitation because it opened the door to cross-contamination. . . .[29]

In the case *Commission v. France* (C-1/00), the European Court of Justice ultimately ruled against France's unilateral ban on UK beef and cattle products, arguing that France was in violation of its obligations as a member of the European Union. Other European countries (including Russia, Spain, Poland, and Hungary) announced in November 2000 that they would place total or partial bans on French beef and cattle exports. Germany also saw political fallout and government instability as a result of the crisis: "One key minister was forced to resign, and the government moved quickly to establish a new federal food safety agency."[30]

It becomes possible to think of BSE as an externality or a "public bad"[31] originally generated within the United Kingdom and ultimately disseminated through the exporting of MBM feed and live cattle to the rest of the world. In this sense BSE may be seen as a global public bad akin to HIV and SARS, with specific geographic and customary origins, transmitted across the globe through complex vectors of transmission. Fox elaborates:

Infected animals from the UK were detected in Canada, Oman, and the Falkland Islands, in addition to six European countries. Exports of MBM from the UK ... reach(ed) approximately 15,000 tons ... in 1988. Most went to EU countries but some also went ... to non-EU countries including Indonesia, Thailand and Sri Lanka. As a result of the ruminant feed ban in the UK, exports to the EU and other countries doubled between 1988 and 1989. When EU countries banned MBM from the UK or introduced their own feed bans in 1989, exports to non-EU countries increased. ... It appears that until the mid 1990s, potentially infective MBM from the UK continued to be exported to countries that did not have ruminant feed bans.[32]

Messerlin has argued that the European Union's Common Agricultural Policy (CAP) may have been partially to blame for the spread of the BSE agent throughout EU countries. In this sense, then, BSE is

a derivative of the CAP, which has induced French (and European) farmers to shift resources away from unprotected soja (protein-rich) crops to highly protected cereals, beef, and sheep. In order to get the amount of proteins needed for improving productivity in milk and meat production, European farmers have often fed their cattle with a by-product—the "meat-and-bone meals" (MBMs)—abundant because European beef production is highly subsidized by the CAP. French MBM producers are linked to slaughterhouses ... enjoying regional monopolies granted by the French state.[33]

Ultimately, the BSE crisis is evidence of a significant regulatory failure for the European Union as well. Krapohl argues that the EU's capacity to regulate during the crisis was effectively blocked by the particular economic and political interests of the member states.[34] "Until 1996," Krapohl notes elsewhere, "common regulations were prevented because British interests dominated the Scientific Veterinary Committee, the committee that advised the Commission on these matters, and played down the dangers of BSE for human health. ... That failure was deemed to be corrected by the establishment of the ... Scientific Steering Committee.

However, the regulations proposed by this committee were blocked by the member states in the Standing Veterinary Committee. . . ."[35]

"The BSE crisis," Messerlin concludes, "provides two lessons. It stresses the urgent need of deep reforms in the European Union. By banning the domestic use of MBMs while allowing their exports to the European Union, Britain has not fully integrated the co-sovereignty dimension implicit in the EU. Meanwhile, by bashing Britain without imposing adequate measures on their own producers in a timely fashion, the other EU member-states have not exerted their own sovereignty."[36]

As per the British domestic experience, the BSE crisis damaged citizens' perceptions of the regulatory efficacy of EU institutions, and undermined the perceived legitimacy of EU scientific bodies, who discounted the probability of the pathogen's proliferation beyond the borders of the United Kingdom. Again, at the EU level, the crisis proved catalytic and opened a temporal window for the reformation of EU institutions. Echoing Schumpeter once more, the crisis did in fact create a brief window of transformation of the EU bureaucracy, in that it allowed for the formation of the European Food Safety Authority in 2002.[37] Furthermore, as a direct result of the crisis the European Union established a Directorate General for Health and Consumer Affairs. However, there is no comprehensive European health policy to speak of.

The BSE crisis also temporarily damaged relations between the European Union, its member states, and other countries. One interesting example is that of Saudi Arabia, which banned beef and mutton products from the EU on January 7, 2001. The Saudi Commerce Ministry expressed its grave concern with EU practices, arguing that "cheating and collusion" had occurred within the bureaucracies in certain EU states to facilitate the export of tainted products from the United Kingdom to developing countries.[38] Moreover, the persistent problems associated with BSE have complicated relations between the European Union and the United States on a number of matters, including trade in hormone-free beef. Specifically, the outbreaks of Mad Cow Disease, and subsequently foot-and-mouth disease in several EU countries, laid the groundwork to impede any resolution of the persistent meat hormone dispute between Brussels and Washington. "The EU," Raymond Ahearn noted in 2005, "has recently indicated its intention to make the ban on hormone-treated meat permanent. . . . In discussions held June 11, 2001, a US industry proposal for expanded access to the EU market for hormone-free beef for a period of 12 years was rejected by the EU. The compensation talks have since languished."[39]

Prions in North America

In 2001, a report by the Harvard Center for Risk Analysis made the bold claim that "BSE is extremely unlikely to be established in the US," echoing the assurances made to citizens by British scientists, and subsequently by the cognoscenti of the European Union.[40] Unfortunately, such assessments of risk were again proved inaccurate. William Leiss argues that by focusing exclusively on the threat that Transmissible Spongiform Encephalopathies (TSEs) posed to human health, such studies erred by ignoring the profound economic risks associated with the discovery of just a few cases of prion-induced disease in North American cattle stocks.[41] In May 2003, the discovery of a single case of BSE in Alberta resulted in an immediate embargo on Canadian cattle and beef exports, and lost markets in the lucrative markets of the United States, Japan, Mexico, and South Korea.[42] With the revelation that BSE had made its way to North American cattle stocks, the US Department of Agriculture immediately banned all imports of Canadian beef, cattle products, and ruminants. As Canadian safeguards were subsequently enacted, the USDA announced the resumption of imports in October 2003.[43] The discovery of the first American case (in December 2003, in the state of Washington) generated moderately destructive effects on the US industry as well.

In the wake of the revelation of BSE's introduction to North America, it is important to contrast the various negative effects on Canada with those experienced by the United States. O'Neill notes that "within days of the USDA's announcement on December 23, 2003, eighteen countries has closed their borders to US beef imports. In total, the United States lost access to seventy overseas markets. However, by way of contrast, only 10 percent of US beef and cattle are exported."[44] Because of the United States' relatively limited dependence on export revenues, as compared to Canada, the economic fallout from the crisis was limited. After the discovery of this first case of BSE in the United States, the US federal government commissioned a study by an International Review Team to analyze the efficacy of the domestic response. While the IRT determined that the US response was generally adequate in a rudimentary sense, it recommended additional actions, including a comprehensive national

BSE surveillance program. The USDA declined to adopt such policies, citing significant costs. However, the decision to circumscribe surveillance efforts is doubtless the result of those domestic stakeholder groups and other pro-business factions who have profound influence on USDA policy.

As the ban on Canadian cattle exports persisted, it proved highly destructive to the Canadian cattle industry, which had relied for some time on US facilities for the processing of cattle. The Ranchers-Cattlemen Action Legal Fund and the United Stockgrowers of America obtained an injunction against imports of Canadian products, courtesy of a ruling by US District Court Justice Richard Cebull on April 26, 2004.[45] In September 2004, the international polemics began in earnest. Canadian opposition leader Stephen Harper accused the United States of protectionism. On January 4, 2005, in response to the ruling by Justice Cebull, the USDA issued a formal rule to reopen the border to trade in Canadian beef and cattle products. Litigation continued until the US Court of Appeals for the Ninth Circuit overruled the lower court's original decision in July 2005.[46] Canadian cattle shipments to the United States resumed on July 18, 2005.[47] In February of that year, the USDA's Inspector General had issued a conclusive report that was highly critical of the USDA bureaucracy, stating that the department's actions regarding Canada were "arbitrary and undocumented, policy decisions were poorly communicated to the public (and within the bureaucracy), and controls over the regulatory process were inadequate."[48]

As of January 2006, BSE had been reported in only five cattle that had been bred and raised in North America. However, as the year progressed, the illness appeared to expand. Six new cases were diagnosed in North America, five in Canada and one in the United States. Although authorities in Ottawa and in Washington suggest that most of these new cases were born before the 1997 feed ban came into effect, this has yet to be conclusively determined.[49] Under pressure from the Western provinces, which were hurt by the economic loss resulting from U.S. embargo, the federal government in Ottawa was forced to intervene, providing more than $C1.4 billion in aid to offset the losses.[50] Unfortunately for Canada, a new case of BSE was confirmed on February 7, 2007, leading to another round of strident criticism by US domestic producers and to demands that the border be closed and that a systematic (and effective) tracking system of cattle be implemented. It would appear that Ottawa is experiencing continuing difficulties in enforcing domestic compliance with its dictates to stem the expansion of BSE. The US criticism of Ottawa continues, largely spurred by the fact that US domestic interests seek to overturn Asian bans on US cattle exports, particularly that of South Korea. And the persistence of BSE in North America undermines Asian confidence in the safety of US beef.

While it is the fashion to blame Ottawa for the continuing perceptions of North American cattle and beef as tainted, the lack of surveillance in the United States impedes the clarification of the integrity of US stocks and thus only reinforces perceptions that the United States is hiding a greater problem. That in turn translates into continuing suspicions regarding the nature of US cattle stocks (and reinforces domestic fears about the food supply), and those suspicions undermine foreign confidence and lead to continuing impediments for the export of US beef exports to foreign markets such as Japan and South Korea. The inhibition of surveillance efforts by the US cattlemen's association (and its institutional vassal, the USDA) seems paradoxical and irrational, particularly if US beef stocks are in fact safe. Common sense would dictate that, in the context of a clean domestic stock, the various factions that benefit from beef exports would go out of their way to demonstrate the purity of the stocks, and therefore rejuvenate US exports. Naturally, then, the Japanese and others remain wary of US beef exports.

Economic Impact

The BSE-induced loss of export markets for Canada generated significant economic damage, which ranged as high as C$500 million per month. Ottawa subsequently committed C$460 million in compensation to producers injured by the crisis.[51] With greater relative levels of cattle and beef exports to foreign markets, Canada has suffered much more from the embargoes than the United States. O'Neill writes:

Cattle and calf prices dropped almost 50 percent between May and July 2003. . . . Market receipts for cattle and calves in the third quarter of 2003 tumbled to less than $500 m, down 73 percent from the $1.8bn recorded in the third quarter of 2002. From May to December the US was the direct beneficiary of Canada's woes: its exports to the rest of the world increased by 17 percent, more than filling the gap left by the loss of Canada's exports. . . . By the time the USDA eased its ban on Canadian beef imports, it was estimated that the loss of Canada's export trade was costing $C11 million per day, and 5,000 jobs had been lost.[52]

In the United States the cattle industry accounts for circa 20 percent of annual revenues from agricultural production. According to USDA figures, estimated revenues derived from US beef and other cattle products were approximately $3 billion in 2003, and the four primary foreign consumers of US beef are, historically, Japan at 37 percent, South Korea at 24 percent, Mexico at 20 percent, and Canada at 10 percent, collectively accounting for 90 percent of annual US beef exports.[53]

After the discovery of BSE in the United States in 2003, most importers immediately banned the importation of US beef products—including Japan and Korea, which maintained restrictions on US beef exports as of April 2008. As of early 2008, Canada and Mexico have relaxed their bans, with Canada hoping to enjoy reciprocity from Washington. The tarnished image of US beef supplies has resulted in a significant decline in the United States' share of the global beef market, from an estimated 18 percent in 2003 to a mere 3 percent as of late 2005.[54] Specifically, total US beef exports in 2003 (before the BSE scare) were on the order of 2500 million pounds, which subsequently declined in dramatic fashion to a mere 425 million pounds in 2004, a decline of 83 percent. US exports have since rebounded to a modest 1.431 billion pounds in 2007.[55]

Similarly, the abrupt decline in demand for US beef products in 2003 resulted in a dramatic yet relatively short-lived decline in the price of beef, as the average price for slaughter-ready cattle plummeted to about $60.00 in 2003 and much of 2004. Despite the loss of certain foreign markets the price of beef has steadily increased over time to approximately $97.80 as of March 15, 2007.[56]

One 2005 study concluded that BSE-induced losses to the US beef industry from lost exports in 2004 alone ranged from $3.2 billion to $4.7 billion.[57] And according to computations by the US National Cattleman's Association, losses in 2005 amounted to circa $4.7 billion.[58] (See figure 5.1.)

The United States and Canada have adopted similar containment regimes, which include the banning of MBM feeds, limited herd surveillance through randomized testing, and bans of imports from countries known to harbor BSE. But in early 2007 the USDA announced that it was significantly reducing its domestic BSE surveillance program by more than 90 percent and closing several labs around the country. While US cattle producers push their state legislatures to tag and track cattle imported from Canada, they oppose the introduction of a similar system

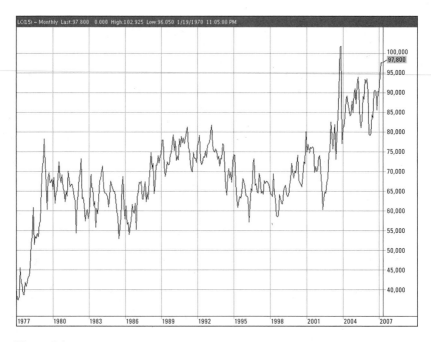

Figure 5.1
Historic cattle prices, annual average, US$, 1977–2007 (CMEX data).

for American cattle.[59] The USDA's opposition to such a system is likely a function of its extensive penetration by domestic stakeholders, which severely limits its autonomy.

In the United States, continuing tensions between the federal government and certain domestic stakeholders who have sought to benefit from the ban have exacerbated relations between Ottawa and Washington over the time period involved. O'Neill notes that the conduct of both governments has been less than rational: "... it is hard to imagine a worse way for the officials of two leading, highly integrated economies to handle this sort of crisis."[60] Of course, the problems between Ottawa and Washington are not nearly as simple as might be assumed, as the game involves a number of players, including Tokyo and Seoul. Specifically, the lack of agreement among Japan, South Korea, and the United States directly results in the persistence of the ban on Canadian stocks, as the continuing occurrences of BSE in North America affect Asian perceptions of the safety of American beef and cattle stocks. This emanates from the accurate perception by Asian export markets that the

Canadian and US cattle and beef industries are in fact linked into one macro-level entity.

The BSE crisis has proved somewhat detrimental to US-Japanese cooperation in recent years, notably in the domain of trade. This is odd given that BSE was actually discovered in Japanese cattle stocks on September 10, 2001, predating its emergence in North America. The emergence of BSE in Japan is most likely linked to the importation of tainted cattle or MBM feed from Britain in the mid to late 1990s. Tokyo's announcement of infected domestic stocks sent prices of Japanese cattle into a tailspin, with retail prices declining to circa 40–50 percent below the levels seen in 2000. The crisis also reduced Japanese demand for imported beef, with US exports to Japan declining by 42 percent in the first two quarters of 2002, well before the discovery of BSE in US stocks.[61]

The persistent Japanese (and South Korean) wariness of US stocks has complicated attempts to resolve the long-standing dispute between Washington and Ottawa. The Japanese have insisted that the United States institute a cattle and beef product tracing program that identifies each animal's place of origin. Adding to the complexities of the situation, Tokyo also has explicitly included "the provision that the United States not lift its ban on Canadian imports" before Japan agrees to normalize trade relations with the United States on this matter.[62] In October 2004, the United States and Japan developed a framework for re-opening trade in beef between the two countries. Trade in beef products briefly resumed in December 2005 until Tokyo discovered vertebrae in US exports, whereupon the ban on US beef products was reinstated. In July 2006, Japan opened its market once again to US beef exports. and trade has resumed. Japanese skepticism of the safety of US exports, and their persistent refusal to re-open their market to US products, has resulted in retaliatory proposals in the US Congress from 2003 to 2006, particularly S.1922/H.R.4179, which proposed $3.14 billion in retaliatory tariffs against Tokyo unless it dropped its ban.

The BSE crisis has certainly damaged the Japanese people's perceptions of the safety and desirability of beef, and of North American beef in particular. According to Becker, perceptions of North American food safety are so poor that "many Japanese consumers (and some officials there) reportedly remain opposed to resuming US imports regardless of whether the government clears the way for them. Meanwhile, these consumers have been substituting other proteins (i.e. pork) and other beef sources (i.e. Australia and New Zealand) for US beef, which once

accounted for 25–30 percent of Japanese beef consumption."[63] The negative implications of the BSE pandemic are certainly not lost on senior US
government officials. Ostfield has noted that high levels of uncertainty
regarding prions induced significant levels of fear, which then subsequently generated significant economic damage to stakeholders in the
United States:

> The psychological effects on consumer behavior as a result of fear and anxiety
> over the possibility of a contaminated food product (loss in consumer confidence)
> can also have a ripple effect on other aspects of the economy. This problem is
> not exclusive to the US. Given Europe's experience with natural outbreaks of
> [BSE]. . . . European officials are acutely aware of the potential impact . . . shorter
> term economic cost, permanent market loss, and potential political fall-
> out. . . . While the human death toll from CJD in the UK was relatively low (158),
> the linkage between BSE and human health led to international bans of British
> beef imports, depressed markets for British beef, crippled the UK's cattle indus-
> try, and destroyed consumer confidence in the UK's ability to handle a health
> and agriculture threat.[64]

Trade between the United States and South Korea has also seen
increased tensions over the BSE affair. Seoul recently vowed to maintain
its quarantine of US beef after recent imports had been found to contain
minute bone chips. There is some evidence that the United States is trying
to link Korean permission for imports containing small bone chips to
the passage of a Free Trade Agreement between the two parties. As of
early 2007 such attempts to mollify the Korean public and improve
perceptions of the safety of US beef had been relatively unsuccessful. In
February 2007, Korean farmers launched protests to block the admission
of such US beef products into the Korean food supply. However, as of
April 2008 US beef exports were penetrating the Korean market.[65]

On Risk, Perception, Emotion, and Cognition

Setbon et al. confirm that risk perception is best described by a model
that incorporates "the importance of feelings and the impossibility
or reducing perceived risk to its cognitive dimension."[66] Such a "hot-
cognitive" model posits that psychological processes of cognition are in
fact subject to various constraints, such as affect or emotion, that may
impede rationality. The political psychologist David Redlawsk concurs,
and posits that "affective biases may easily lead to lower quality decision
making, leading to direct challenges to the notion of (humans) as rational

Bayesian updaters."[67] Echoing such concerns regarding the irrationality of responses by affected countries, the Organization for Animal Health has argued that policy makers tend to overreact and impose draconian trade embargoes without conducting a sober and rational science-based risk analysis of the threat posed by BSE.

Theoretical Ramifications

The empirical destruction of human life from Variant Creutzfeld-Jacob Disease has in fact proved to be rather minimal, certainly as compared to banes such as the global HIV/AIDS pandemic. One might note that the destruction wrought by the epizootic BSE has proven to be empirically quite devastating to herds of cattle, originally in the United Kingdom, and ultimately throughout the European Union. This ultimately serves to reinforce psychological analysis of the BSE pandemic. In this case, extreme levels of uncertainty regarding modes of transmission, the likelihood of becoming infected, and the slow and horrid death associated with VCJD all combined to generate exceptional levels of fear in the general population. Such high levels of affect only served to exacerbate the economic damage done by the spread of the disease, as panic served to destabilize markets. Ergo, the affective psychological component (fear, anxiety) associated with this form of contagion is of exceptional significance. This reinforces political psychology arguments which hold that perception, cognition, and affect may generate suboptimal outcomes, which in this case resulted in serious deviations from rationality.

The persistent overreaction of societies, and lack of effective reaction by sovereign states may not only result from a combination of affective bias coupled with the predominance of the precautionary principle; it may also be attributable to the fact that the "scientific experts" have been proved wrong time and again, in Britain, throughout the European Union, in Japan, and in North America. The political scientist Peter Haas espoused the notion that "epistemic communities" functioned as effective agents of positive change, with the scientist functioning as political agent.[68] In fact, "epistemic communities" have been shown to be persistently in error throughout the attenuated BSE crisis. Moreover, scientists have also been perceived as the vassals of corporate interests and government bureaucracies, and dismissive of the public interest writ large. Collectively, then, public perceptions of the legitimacy of epistemic communities have declined. Thus, another long-term repercussion of the BSE scare, particularly in Europe, is the lingering mistrust of "expert opinion" in general, and of genetically modified foods in particular. "Expert assurances," Robert Paarlberg argues, "are discounted by European consumers, distrustful since the 1996 'mad cow disease' scare. That crisis undermined consumer trust in expert opinion after UK public health officials gave consumers what proved to be a false assurance that there was no danger in eating beef from diseased animals. Although mad cow disease had nothing to do with the genetic modification of food, it generated new anxieties about food safety"[69] as GM products were being introduced to the EU market. Thus, the BSE epizootic is associated with negative effects on public perceptions of the legitimacy of epistemic communities, as the scientific community became perceived as either incompetent, or as corrupt and beholden to the private sector. This decline in legitimacy is unusual given the historical successes of epistemic communities in promoting the protection and remediation of complex ecological systems,[70] or in the promotion of controls to inhibit the proliferation of nuclear weapons.[71] Therefore, the case of the BSE epizootic provides a powerful exception to the rule of epistemic communities functioning as benign and effective agents of positive change in the realm of the political. Moreover, this case provides yet another sober look at the limited capacity of epistemic communities to accurately assess risk when faced with an emergent pathogen, and then to collaborate effectively with state institutions to mitigate that threat. Furthermore, the case of BSE raises the possibility of rivalrous epistemic communities, as espoused by the political scientist Jeremy Youde.[72] In this case, those scientists in the employ of the agri-business factions and cattlemen's lobby in the United States, faced off against scientists in the USDA, who in turn were pitted against their counterparts in Ottawa, casting doubt on the Haasian notion of the unified and autonomous epistemic community acting free of bias. Therefore, I argue that it is in fact expedient to take Youde's formulation a step further, and to postulate the fragmentation of epistemic communities, and/or the existence of multiple rivalrous epistemic communities, each serving their various embedded interests and reflecting those biases, echoing the problems witnessed during our examinations of the response to SARS and to HIV/AIDS.

The BSE crisis also served to undermine the perceived legitimacy of those institutions of governance, both at the domestic and inter-state level, that were involved in the diagnosis and control of the pathogen.

Public confidence in the integrity of the institutions involved has declined significantly, particularly in Europe, as a result of the BSE affair. On an institutional level, this case also provides additional support for the concept of contagion as a catalytic agent that provides an opportunity for Schumpeterian notions of "creative destruction," wherein ineffective institutions (such as the MAFF in the United Kingdom) were dismantled and replaced by increasingly effective institutions. In this way, disease is not so much viewed as apocalyptic, but rather as transformative, providing a window of opportunity for important institutional reformation, both at the domestic and to a lesser extent at the supra-national level. Within the North American context the emergence of BSE generated considerable domestic and foreign concern over the safety of the US and Canadian food supplies, and the protection of public health. Both Canadian and US beef markets have suffered from a loss of confidence in their integrity, and a loss of confidence in the institutions designed to protect that integrity. However, the relatively minor nature of the epizootic (and in the incidence of human disease) in North America has not led to any major institutional reformation in the United States, while it provided impetus to affect a degree of institutional change in the Canadian case, namely the creation of the Public Health Agency of Canada in 2004.

In addition, the BSE crisis has illuminated the shortcomings of Marxist explanations of disease prevalence, which hold that poverty, and the global maldistribution of wealth explain all patterns of disease incidence and pathogenic emergence. As documented above, the wealthy state of Britain (a member of the G-8 no less) served as the global epicenter of the emerging BSE crisis, with the contagion ultimately spreading to more than 23 countries. This is crucial, in that a new zoonosis originated not in the developing countries, but rather in a wealthy and technically sophisticated member of the European Union. Moreover, the contagion spread from the United Kingdom to the other wealthy and technologically sophisticated countries of the European Union, and subsequently to Canada, the United States, and Japan. Thus, emergent infections are not in fact solely a function of the global distribution of wealth, as reductionists in the Marxist school would have us believe, but rather that pathogens evolve in complex fashion to fill ecological niches within all societies. The emergence of other pathogens within the context of wealthy and developed societies helps to illustrate this concept, ranging from *Legionella* in air conditioning systems to antibiotic resistant diseases such as

MRSA and VRE, which have colonized the North American hospital systems. As was noted above, the SARS epidemic is yet another powerful example of a modern global epidemic that resulted from zoonosis and thrived in the nosocomial ecologies of modern industrial societies.

On balance, international cooperation has proved to be rather problematic in the face of the BSE pandemic. Relations between sovereign states have been marred by polemics, a series of painful trade embargoes, and some limited disruption of a supra-national organization such as the European Union, and inter-state accords such as NAFTA. Ultimately, the BSE-induced discord that persists between many countries offsets the nascent cooperation that has begun to occur in the European Union. On a theoretical level, this case casts considerable doubt on liberal institutional models of international relations, which predict cooperation between sovereign states, and reinforces elements of republican Realist paradigm which stresses the protection of perceived self-interest, and territorial sovereignty, and predicts competitive behavior between states. O'Neill concurs: "... when public health is threatened by "foreign" diseases, countries almost always act first by protecting their borders."[73] The constructive facet of the paradigm also predicts that states do not adhere to the Rational Actor Model, which "views decision making as a utility—or value—maximizing process."[74] The Pareto-suboptimal decision making that has characterized the BSE issue suggests that both conventional Realist and Liberal theory is in need of some refinement, particularly in their inabilities to explain such irrational mistakes in foreign policy decision making.[75] While the European Union has finally obtained some form of cohesion on the issue, the initially obstructionist responses by Britain, France, and other sovereign states within the union gives additional credibility to the republican Realist model. Furthermore, the continuing lack of effective cooperation between Ottawa and Washington, and the inability of the NAFTA states to gain cooperation from their Asian partners, suggests that Pareto-suboptimal irrationality, coupled with unenlightened self-interest, and tendencies toward protectionism are the norm in this case. Collectively such behavior provides preliminary evidence that undermines the validity of the neo-liberal model which privileges cooperation and rationality. Moreover, neo-liberal theorists hold that international institutions would be highly effective in facilitating cooperation between sovereign states, and yet the BSE case indicates that the efficacy of international organizations is weak at best. In the case of the European Union it experienced many years of pronounced discord between its member states, and had to use coercion (through threat of legal sanctions) to get its members to comply with EU statutes. NAFTA has been largely ineffective as a means of resolving the ongoing disputes between the United States and Canada, and international organizations (such as the WTO and the G-8) have shown themselves to be equally ineffective in resolving the disputes between the North American and Asian states. Collectively, the evidence to date suggests that orthodox liberal theory has a rather difficult time in explaining the international acrimony generated by the BSE affair.

Globalization and recent advances in communications technologies have amplified the effects of this epizootic. BSE-induced uncertainty, fear, and anxiety have been transmitted via the mass media across the globe, resulting in the intensification of the affective response, and undermining the ability to assess risk which in turn leads to overreaction. Perversely then, the processes of globalization, such as increased trade, global markets in commodities, the increased flows of information via global media have all contributed to the emergence of this global "public bad" or externality. In a sense, then, the BSE crisis exhibits emergent properties as well, as changes in animal husbandry, leading to prion emergence, combined with such aforementioned processes of globalization to generate the profound levels of fear and uncertainty that ultimately inflicted significant economic damage on affected countries, and generated protracted political discord between sovereign states.

Moreover, the symbolic nature of the BSE crisis reinforces republican theory. The emergence of BSE was seen as resulting from human violations of the laws of nature, of modern "progress" gone horribly awry as cows were converted into carnivores to enrich certain economic factions of society. This symbolism reinforces perceptions of BSE as a plague-like visitation on humanity, as a form of almost divine retribution, and as punishment for the violation of natural law. Such notions of punishment for violations of the natural order has led to the search for "the other" as scapegoat. Whether the other is the government, cattle producers, or foreign peoples, the perception of the other as being culpable (and therefore the progenitor of the plague) is widespread, and undermines the capacity for cooperation between affected parties.

The processes of scapegoating, of constructing the other as the guilty party, so prevalent over the broad span of history, appears to persist in this case as well. Fisher comments:

A striking characteristic of the historical reaction to plagues has been the pervasive belief that they are a form of retribution exacted for the sins or failings of society and that these sins or failings can be expiated through the punishment of offenders. . . . As the state took on the responsibility for the execution of policies designed to contain or eradicate plagues, it and its agencies became a logical target in the case of perceived failure.[76]

In sum, the BSE case illustrates the utility of combining Realist perspectives that emphasize self-interest and competitive anarchy, with those elements of Constructivism that focus on perception and cognition, particularly within an affect-laden hot-cognition model wherein affect may generate significant deviations from rationality. The republican Realist model incorporates elements of both Realism and political psychology, given that they are both descendants of republican theory. The case also illustrates the problems latent in the literature on epistemic communities, as rivalrous factions of epistemic communities occur in this case, and epistemic communities (with their continued inability to assess the risks) are often no longer perceived as competent by the people. Moreover the difficulties in risk assessment and containment, so evident in the European and North American cases, have also served to undermine the perceptions of the legitimacy of state institutions, particularly in the European context.

Epidemic of Fear: SARS and the Political Economy of Contagion in the Pacific Rim

The SARS epidemic of 2002–03 provides another glimpse into the significance of emergent infectious disease as an agent of destabilization at both the domestic and international levels. During this outbreak, SARS generated significant levels of fear and psychological trauma in affected populations, impeded international trade and migration flows, and resulted in minor to moderate economic damage to the economies of affected Pacific Rim countries (particularly China and Canada). In this chapter, I argue that while the SARS epidemic may have generated moderate institutional change at the domestic level (particularly in China and Canada), it resulted in only ephemeral change at the level of global governance. In the domain of security, I argue that despite minor demographic effects, the epidemic generated moderate levels of fear-induced economic damage that constituted a direct threat to the material interests of affected states, particularly China, Hong Kong, and Singapore. Moreover, the epidemic possessed the potential to evolve into a global pandemic that might have generated much greater loss of life and economic damage, and thereby constituted a threat to international security.

Demographic Impact and Etiology

Despite the fact that the SARS epidemic threatened the prosperity of seriously affected countries, and posed a grave threat to the health of populations in the region, it was successfully contained with relatively little mortality. Specifically, the epidemic resulted in 8,096 cases of infection (morbidity) and 774 deaths (mortality) between November 1, 2002 and August 7, 2003,[1] exhibiting a mortality rate of approximately 10.88 percent of those infected. The SARS coronavirus is a novel zoonosis that recently crossed over from its natural animal reservoirs into the human ecology, presumably in late 2002.[2] Specifically, the SARS coronavirus resides in bat populations in Southeast Asia,[3] which bite and transmit the virus to palm civets (*Paguma larvata*), whereupon strains that infect civets possess a greater capacity to then infect individual humans and thereafter become endogenized within the human ecology.[4]

The moderate level of economic damage generated by the epidemic was not so much the result of the (relatively minor) morbidity and mortality that SARS induced, but emanated from the pernicious psychological effects (fear, anxiety, and panic) that the epidemic generated,[5] both within infected areas and in uninfected populations. These significant levels of affect resulted in suboptimal economic outcomes for the entire Pacific Rim as tourism ground to halt, international trade flows were slowed, and foreign investors cautiously withdrew capital from the region during the crisis.

Background

Literature on the political dimensions of the epidemic remains exceedingly sparse. The microbiologist Elizabeth Prescott argued that the SARS epidemic illustrates the increasingly acute nature of complex interdependence among countries in the domain of public health, and provides us with lessons that may help countries in their efforts to prevent bioterrorist attacks. She observed that the emergence of the contagion "illuminated significant and vital weaknesses in global and local preparedness for surprise outbreaks."[6] The political scientists Melissa Curley and Nicholas Thomas argued that infectious diseases (the SARS outbreak in particular) represented a significant and growing threat to human security in Southeast Asia. The legal scholar David Fidler has also conceptualized SARS as a threat to the material interests of the state, which aligns with the republican Realist model presented in this work.[7] The emergence of the SARS pathogen in China and later in Canada demonstrates that both developing and highly developed countries remain vulnerable to emerging and re-emerging pathogens. Despite the (erroneous) Galenic notion that infectious disease arises solely from and within poor countries, and is only a scourge of the poor, SARS illustrates that disease is not simply a product of the inequitable distribution of wealth. In reality, SARS emerged to take advantage of specific changes in the relationship between its natural reservoirs and the human ecology of

Southeast Asia. Its proliferation in Hong Kong, Singapore, and Toronto and illustrates the principal that developed countries are not immune to the deleterious effects of novel epidemic disease agents.

History

According to the political scientist Yanzhong Huang, the first SARS case "is thought to have occurred in Foshan, a city southwest of Guangzhou in Guangdong province, in mid November 2002."[8] The index case was the physician Liu Jianlun, who inadvertently fomented a global chain of transmission when he traveled to Hong Kong and stayed at the now infamous Metropole Hotel. Liu then infected other travelers who subsequently spread the disease throughout the Pacific Rim countries. On March 12, 2003, the World Health Organization issued a global outbreak alert and initiated international surveillance efforts to track the contagion. By that point the pathogen had spread throughout the countries of the Pacific Rim, with the greatest incidence of cases in China (5,327), followed by Hong Kong (1,755), Taiwan (665), Canada (251), Singapore (238), Vietnam (63), and the United States (33), respectively.[9]

Effective response to the epidemic was initially compromised by both psychological factors (fear, confusion, and denial) and bureaucratic ineptitude and corruption in China. Political elites in Guangzhou and Beijing conspired in a deliberate attempt to suppress knowledge of the epidemic in both the domestic and international arenas. Health officials in Beijing ordered that reports on the proliferation of the pathogen be classified as "top secret," such that the disclosure or discussion of the outbreak constituted a direct violation of national secrets.[10] The burgeoning epidemic generated profound levels of fear among the general Chinese population and warnings about the virus filtered out to the global community via the Internet. Despite such leaks, Beijing persisted in its attempts to mislead the WHO, as on February 27 the Chinese Ministry of Health declared the epidemic to be officially contained. In fact the disease continued its rapid proliferation throughout the population of Beijing.[11] The Chinese façade disintegrated on April 4, when the head of China's Center for Disease Control publicly apologized to the Chinese people, and to the international community, for failing to inform the public about a highly contagious and often lethal new pathogen.[12] The full extent of Beijing's duplicity became clear on April 9, when Jiang

Yanyong, a prominent member of the Communist Party (and a physician), publicly accused the government of covering up the extent of the epidemic in Beijing.[13]

On April 16 the WHO took the unprecedented step of publicly chastising Beijing for misleading the global community as to the true extent of SARS infection throughout that country.[14] Two days later Beijing announced a national "war" on the virus, and ordered all Communist Party officials to reveal the true extent of the epidemic or be held accountable for their deliberate obfuscation. On April 2), the Party leadership demanded the resignation of the Minister of Health, Zhang Wenkang, and the Mayor of Beijing, Meng Xuenong, for their complicity in the conspiracy.[15] This move was seen as an attempt to deflect blame from senior party officials for their role in the crisis. On July 5, 2003, the WHO announced that the SARS epidemic had been effectively contained. Despite the fact that the international community successfully contained the spread of the virus in a relatively brief span of time, the medical community insists that it represented a significant global threat. The physician Thomas Tsang commented: "I think there was a possibility of being a global pandemic if the appropriate control measures were not taken."[16]

Psychological Impacts

As was argued above, contagion is historically associated with generating profound levels of affect (i.e. fear and anxiety) within affected populations, particularly in the face of a novel pathogen which generates great uncertainty and inhibits effective risk assessment. Uncertainty and fear result in suboptimal decision making which may in turn result in very real damage to a country's material interests. The SARS epidemic provides a vivid illustration of this dynamic, as the emergence of the novel, virulent, and transmissible SARS coronavirus generated profound levels of anxiety and significant economic damage throughout the countries of the Pacific Rim. This fear was compounded by the fact that public health officials originally suspected that SARS might be a novel and virulent strain of influenza.

As a novel pathogen, SARS presented an enigma to public health personnel who were largely unaware of the symptoms, routes of transmission and effective prevention of transmission during its outbreak. This uncertainty resulted in diagnostic delays, misdiagnosis, and also put health-care workers at considerable risk. Infected health-care providers infected accounted for 21 percent of all cases, ranging from a mere 3 percent of reported probable cases in the United States to 43 percent in Canada. Witnessing that nurses and doctors were unable to protect themselves from the infection, the public developed a highly exaggerated estimate of their personal risk of being infected. Surveys conducted in Hong Kong during the period of contagion indicate that respondents experienced profound levels of negative affect, and psychological stress, as a result of the contagion.[17] Echoing the contagionist responses of the past, Beijing's draconian measures to control the flow of information, and persistent delays in reporting data, only served to magnify the levels of fear and anxiety afflicting the general population. By late April 2003, in a replay of the contagion-induced flights so common in the years of plague and cholera, an estimated million people (about 10 percent of the population) had fled Beijing for other parts of China.[18] They would soon find themselves unwelcome even in their hometowns, perceived as vectors of pathogen transmission. In the countryside, worried villagers set up roadblocks to restrict the entry of refugees from Beijing, and a series of riots against rural quarantine centers were also reported in May 2003.[19]

Economic Impacts

China

The profound levels of epidemic-induced fear resulted in substantial negative economic impacts on affected countries, although such impacts were brief. The transmissibility of the pathogen, and the perceived risk of exposure through social interaction, induced significant behavioral change in affected populations. Consonant with the historical experience of influenza, social distancing techniques were utilized and people were cajoled into avoiding mass gatherings in public places. Moreover, the fear of contagion and the implementation of anti-epidemic measures also discouraged travel and interrupted transport services, inducing substantial declines in consumer demand, particularly in the service sector. Such adverse demand-induced shocks affected two industries in particular: retail sales and tourism. By mid April 2003, retail sales in Hong Kong had declined by 50 percent relative to mid-March indicators. Additionally, tourism arrivals from mainland China had declined by 75–80 percent, and the entertainment and restaurant industries had recorded an 80 percent decline in business. In general, the economic shock was far greater for those economies with a prominent service sector and which possessed a larger share of impacted industries (i.e., retail sale and tourism) within that sector. This may explain why Hong Kong, with its losses accounting for 2.9 percent of GDP, suffered the worst. In early April 2003, Stephan Roach, an economist with the firm Morgan Stanley, estimated the global economic cost of SARS at circa US$30 billion.[20] The *Far Eastern Economic Review* later estimated initial SARS-related damage to regional GDP growth at US$10.6–15 billion. If SARS had continued to spread, quarantines could have affected manufacturing, which accounts for approximately 30 percent of Asia's GDP (minus Japan), by closing factories and slowing trade. If the costs of premature deaths of income-earners, lost workdays of sick employees, and health care were factored into the equation, the eventual bill for the region could total almost $50 billion.[21]

China sustained significant losses in its service sector, which makes up 33.7 percent of the country's GDP. SARS caused a decline in sectoral productivity of 6.8 percent during the second quarter. According to a government economist, the loss borne by the sector was 23.5 billion yuan, including 20 billion in tourism and 3.5 billion in retail sales. Based on the economic indicators of China's economy affected by SARS, the Asian Development Bank put the GDP losses in China at US$6.1 billion, or 0.5 percent of total GDP. If calculated by total final expenditure, the total loss is 17.9 billion, or 1.3 percent of China's GDP.

Aside from SARS-induced disruptions in the tourism and retail sectors, the fear-induced hoarding of essential goods and currency threatened fiscal liquidity. Moreover, calls by other countries for the quarantine of Chinese goods threatened China's export-driven manufacturing sector. If SARS had persisted and resulted in the disruption the production and supply chains, the increased risk profile associated with doing business in China would have led to a reduction in foreign investment and exports, damaging China's manufacturing sector. The end result would be a decline in the economic growth rate, on which the regime's legitimacy hinges.

Canada

The SARS epidemic generated moderate damage to the Canadian economy, but this damage was brief. At the sectoral level, the SARS epidemic had a pronounced negative effect on the Canadian economy in the second and third quarters of 2003. Industries that bore the brunt of the contagion included tourism and hospitality, and the film industry. Toronto's billion-dollar-a-year film, television, and commercial business was badly damaged by the epidemic of 2003, as foreign production houses withdrew their operations from the city. According to Joe Halstead, then Toronto's commissioner of economic development, the SARS epidemic resulted in a decline of production, resulting in a loss of $163 million (roughly 18 percent) for the film sector in 2003. Commercial production in the city exhibited a similar decline of $32.8 million in 2003 (roughly 20 percent).[22] These statistics were compiled from permit applications that production houses must file with the City of Toronto. Tourism in Ontario also took a significant hit as a result of the epidemic, with Toronto witnessing an estimated a decline of 18 percent during 2003, largely as a function of the epidemic and its aftereffects.[23] According to Jeff Dover of KPMG, the SARS epidemic resulted in the loss of approximately C$993 million in the Tourism sector of the Canadian economy during the second and third quarters of 2003.[24]

On the macro level, SARS seems to have been largely responsible for a pronounced economic downturn in the Province of Ontario, where it resulted in two consecutive quarters of economic decline in 2003. Ontario Finance Minister Gregory Sorbara noted that the widespread decline was "an economic downturn that was driven by SARS."[25] According to Finance Ministry estimates, Ontario's real GDP fell by 0.7 percent in the second quarter of 2003, and by a further 2.5 percent in the third quarter. The economy rebounded in the fourth quarter, when growth reportedly increased by 4.5 percent.[26] The Minister of Health for Ontario during the epidemic, Tony Clement, revealed that SARS had cost the province's health-care system $945 million as of June 27, 2003. Cost increases were associated with extra staffing needs, special supplies required to protect health-care workers, and expenditures to build specialized SARS isolation and treatment facilities.[27] The best estimate is that the contagion cost Ontario at least C$1.5 billion in 2003.

Global SARS-induced economic damage in 2003 amounted to US$40–50 billion. This seems relatively minute compared to the multi-trillion-dollar global economy; however, the damage becomes more apparent when it is stated in terms of a loss to the annual GDP of a given country. The economists Lee and McKibben analyzed the effects of the epidemic, and their most conservative models estimated that SARS generated a 2.6 percent decline in GDP for Hong Kong, and a 1.1 percent decline for mainland China, during 2003.[28] The Asian Development Bank estimated that SARS induced a 1.1 percent decline in GDP per annum for Singapore as well in the most conservative scenario.[29] Those figures represent a significant drag on economic productivity per annum for those affected countries, and therefore we may conclude that SARS constituted a substantive threat to the material interests of those countries.

Effects on Governance

Canada

While the epidemic inflicted significant short-term economic damage to Pacific Rim economies, it also has important implications for intra-state governance. The SARS epidemic revealed significant problems in governance within those sovereign states most affected by the epidemic (Canada and China). The effects of the contagion on governance in Canada, and the dubious responses of the government at both the provincial and the federal level deserve serious investigation. Canada provides a very good example that even a wealthy advanced democracy can experience profound problems in the domain of public health governance. Indeed, SARS revealed the limitations of Ontario's public health-care infrastructure, dramatically eroded by the cuts initiated by the administration of Premier Mike Harris throughout the 1990s, and prompted the federal and provincial governments to review the country's public health policy and infrastructure. The effects of the contagion on governance in Canada, and the questionable responses of the government at both the provincial and federal levels, therefore deserve serious investigation. Specifically, the epidemic revealed that Canada's public health infrastructure was fragile—particularly in the province of Ontario, which saw the most significant outbreak of SARS outside of China. Gambling that budget cuts in public health controls wouldn't matter, in 2001 the of Harris administration laid off five scientists charged with regional disease surveillance.

Ontario experienced significant problems in infection control, ranging from the questionable leadership of Colin D'Cunha, to problems in staffing hospitals, to the persistent violation of quarantine and subsequent spread of infection. The infection of Walkerton's water supply with *E. coli* went unheeded. The Canadian case also illustrates chronic problems in communication between the provincial government in Toronto and the federal government in Ottawa, exacerbated by the perennial conflict over which tier of governance should preside over matters of public health. At present such duties are relegated to the provinces, as is the matter of funding which is supplemented through transfer payments from Ottawa. Partisan differences may have also led the Liberal administration of Prime Minister Jean Chrétien to be less than cooperative with the Conservative administration of Ontario. The Chrétien administration also demonstrated a significant failure of leadership during the crisis. The federal Minister of Health, Ann McClelland, often proved less than cooperative in her dealings with the province and with the World Health Organization. Moreover, Chrétien displayed an appalling lack of leadership when he refused to interrupt his vacation abroad to return to Ottawa and deal with the rapidly expanding epidemic in the Toronto metropolitan area. As a result of these glaring deficiencies in the Canadian response to SARS, several Commissions of Inquiry were commissioned to determine precisely how the system failed, and to develop recommendations for improving the response capacity of Canadian public health delivery.[30]

Prescott chides Canadian officials for their myopic response to the emergence of contagion in Toronto: ". . . Canadian officials appeared to be more concerned with the short-term impact of a (WHO) travel advisory on tourism, retail and other industries, even though the epidemic appeared to have spread through the community and to other countries partially because the Canadian health authorities had ignored a WHO advisory that all departing passengers from Toronto be screened by medical personnel."[31]

Ultimately, the Canadian response to the exogenous shock of the SARS epidemic provides some evidence to confirm the punctuated-equilibrium model. Specifically, in 2004, the Canadian federal government created a new cabinet-level Public Health Agency, led by a Chief Public Health Officer who (despite a certain degree of autonomy) reports to the Minister of Health. A central mission of this nascent agency is to facilitate cooperation between the federal and provincial governments in the domain of public health emergencies. This clearly demonstrates the increasing salience of public health issues in the mind of Canadian political elites. One thing is clear: the SARS debacle has resulted in the elevation of public health to the level of "high politics" in Ottawa. This is evident in the Canadian National Advisory Committee on SARS and Public Health's reference to Benjamin Disraeli's argument that "public health was the foundation for the happiness of the people and the power of the country" and "the care of the public health is the first duty of the statesman."[32] The question is: Can the scientific community sustain the momentum generated by the SARS epidemic to maintain investment in Canadian public health infrastructure, or will political elites revert to the typical human pattern of forgetting about the threat of contagion until the next pathogen arrives?

China

The SARS epidemic exposed significant shortcomings in China's governance structure. Initially, the government chose not to publicize the outbreak for fear that this would have a negative effect on economic development. The suppression of information persisted even after the epidemic spread to Beijing, in part because the party did not want the contagion to disrupt its National People's Congress meeting, a showcase for the Communist Party's highly controlled and carefully staged version of participatory democracy. By April of 2003, it was evident that SARS had captured the attention of the central leadership. However, the formulation of policy to check SARS was impeded by lower-level government officials who manipulated and distorted the flow of information to the higher echelons. Despite the fact that the Ministry of Health was cognizant of a deadly new pneumonia in Guangdong on January 20, 2003; the Chinese Center for Disease Control and Prevention (CDC) did nothing to check the spread of the contagion until April 3. The Chinese government thus waited more than three months before taking decisive action in late April of 2003. Echoing the Canadian case, rivalries existed between various health bureaucracies, territorial governments, and between military and civilian and institutions. Paradoxically, the SARS crisis also granted an opportunity for the Chinese government to address internal governance problems. As Hirschman suggests, politicians have strong incentives to exploit crisis and danger and emphasize the risks of inaction in order to mobilize opinion and arouse action.[33] The political scientist Yanzhong Huang has argued that the legitimacy of the current regime in China is largely performance-based, rooted in delivering economic growth.[34] The possibility of an economic recession caused by SARS, therefore, posed a direct threat to the regime's material interests, and to perceptions of its legitimacy. In the words of Premier Wen Jiaobao, "the health and security of the people, overall state of reform, development, and stability, and China's national interest and international image now are at stake."

The perceived crisis impelled the central leadership to mobilize the state's capacity for containment of the contagion. On April 17, China's leaders convened an urgent meeting to initiate a national campaign to check the spread of the epidemic. This dramatic change in the trajectory of national policy was synchronous with a relaxation of media control as the government publicized the number of SARS cases in each province, with daily updates. Three days later, the Health Minister (Zhang Wenkang) and Beijing's mayor (Meng Xuenong) were ousted for their egregious mismanagement of the crisis. The crisis also precipitated government efforts to increase bureaucratic control and designate greater financial resources for an anti-SARS campaign. On April 23, a task force known as the SARS Control and Prevention Headquarters of the State Council was established to coordinate national efforts to combat the disease, with Vice-Premier Wu Yi appointed as commander-in-chief of the task force. The same day, a national fund of 2 billion yuan (US$242 million) was created for SARS prevention and control. As part of a national campaign to mobilize the apparatus of governance, the State Council sent out inspection teams to 26 provinces to examine government records for unreported cases and to fire officials for lax prevention efforts. According to the official media, by May 8 China had dismissed or penalized more than 120 officials for their ineffective response to the SARS epidemic. These actions energized local government officials, who then abandoned their initial hesitation and jumped onto the anti-SARS bandwagon. In retrospect, the SARS crisis challenged the traditional concept of governance in China and helped to significantly elevate the status of public health on the government's agenda. The government has now realized that economic development does not trickle down, and that public health should be treated as an independent criterion of good governance. Premier Wen Jiabao said that "one important inspirational lesson" the new Chinese leadership learned from the SARS crisis was that any "imbalance between economic development and social development" was "bound to stumble and fall." Huang argues that the government since then has earmarked billions of dollars for the public health sector. More attention has also been paid to the basic needs of the disadvantaged portion of the population, including farmers and workers. The epidemic also created incentives for Chinese leaders to adopt a new, more proactive attitude toward HIV/AIDS. Since then, discourse and action surrounding HIV/AIDS have changed dramatically, with senior leaders facing the epidemic with a greater sense of responsibility.

International

Partially because of the profound economic impact of SARS, partially because of the fear it had created among their citizens, heads of state, diplomats and politicians became involved early and visibly, fully participating in outbreak control through frequent press briefings, declarations, and provision of political and economic support to the global containment effort.

—David Heynmann, in Fidler 2004, p. xiv

As the SARS epidemic intensified, the ten member states of ASEAN (the Association of Southeast Asian Nations) grew increasingly aware of the threat the contagion posed to their people and their economies. Anxiety in this region actually was intensified by earlier shocks to governance in the region, such as the Asian economic crisis of 1997–98, as well as the regional environmental "haze" issue that resulted from ubiquitous fires throughout the region during the same time period. Indeed, fear arose in Singapore that SARS could provoke its worst economic crisis since the country had gained independence.[35] While such concerns over economic loss were shared by leaders in this region, the rapidly spreading epidemic also generated a strong sense of the urgency of regional cooperation. On April 26, the Health Ministers of the ASEAN countries and those of China, Japan, and South Korea met in Kuala Lumpur to voice their willingness to cooperate. On April 29, leaders from the ASEAN countries attended the emergency summit in Bangkok.[36] The Bangkok summit was initiated by Prime Minister Goh Chok Tong of Singapore, who was also instrumental in setting the agenda. ASEAN thus became the ideal platform for discussing this issue. Initiated by Goh, the communiqué issued by Bangkok summit articulated a "collective responsibility to implement stringent measures to control and contain the spread of SARS and the importance of transparency in implementing these measures."[37] ASEAN members agreed that all countries in the region would immediately commence mandatory screening for SARS at their borders. The declaration issued by member states agreed on various measures to stop SARS transmission, including sharing information on the movement of people by building a SARS containment information network, coordinating prevention measures by standardizing health screening for all travelers (i.e., common protocols for air, land, and sea travel), adopting an "isolate and contain" approach (rather than a blank ban on travel), and establishing an *ad hoc* ministerial-level joint task force to follow-up, decide and monitor the implementation of the decisions made at this meeting and the "ASEAN + 3"[38] health ministers' special meeting on SARS.

China and representatives from Hong Kong were invited to attend a follow-up summit later the same day. During that special meeting, however, ASEAN diplomats were very careful not to directly criticize Beijing's mishandling of the epidemic, but rather to solicit China's cooperation in dealing with a highly sensitive issue. The idea was for ASEAN leaders to agree on a set of resolutions and measures for China to sign on to. Aware that the image of the China and the reputation of its new leadership were at stake, Wen was cooperative during the Bangkok conference. He pleaded for understanding from other ASEAN leaders. "In the face of the outbreak of this sudden epidemic," he said, "we lack experience with its prevention and control. The crisis-management mechanism and the work of certain localities and departments are not quite adequate."[39] This was an astonishing admission of culpability from a regime that is loath to admit responsibility for any mistake or wrongdoing. In an ASEAN-China joint statement, China agreed to "associate itself with the measures proposed by the ASEAN declaration." This endorsement by Beijing was indeed remarkable, given that a total embracement of the measures decided by the ASEAN leaders would be perceived in China as an act of submission.[40]

A central problem to pathogen surveillance and containment throughout the region was the dearth of public health infrastructure among many of the poorer countries, an issue of state capacity. To strengthen regional capacity, Beijing provided $1.2 million, subsequently emulated by Thailand and Cambodia.[41] While it was a positive gesture, such meager amounts did not truly generate any significantly increased levels of regional public health infrastructural capacity. Despite the rhetoric of cooperation, containment remained the responsibility of its sovereign member states to implement those principles and to engage in suppression of the contagion.

The political analyst Eric Cheow argues that the fact that the SARS virus developed and emerged in Guangdong province suggests that poverty and low state capacity are the principal variables governing the emergence of infectious disease. "As East Asians develop a sense of community," Cheow writes, "they must look urgently into developing the poorer regions so they will not remain poor, underdeveloped and, thus a hotbed of chronic diseases, which may have been eradicated in the richer and more developed countries."[42] Such assumptions betray a certain degree of ignorance regarding the ecological mechanics of microbial emergence and evolution. As was noted above, selective evolutionary pressures will force microbes to adapt to (and colonize) ecological niches in countries of both high and low state capacity.[43] Ergo, the assumption that the most virulent and transmissible of new pathogens necessarily emanate from the least developed countries (and regions within those countries) is empirically specious.[44]

Moreover, the success of various countries in controlling the epidemic demonstrates that a prosperous country that exhibited significant levels of endogenous capacity (such as Canada) had a much more difficult time in containing the infection than did countries of lower capacity, particularly Vietnam. The most recent epidemiological evidence suggests that SARS appears to thrive under conditions that promote nosocomial transmission.[45] Therefore, the sealed, air-conditioned hospitals of developed societies appeared to facilitate SARS transmission. Conversely, Vietnamese hospitals are often open-aired, diminishing the probability of nosocomial transmission. In other words, the SARS coronavirus appears to be more transmissible in the sealed hospital and urban environments of countries with technologically sophisticated health infrastructures. SARS, then, would seem to pose a greater threat to countries of higher capacity, and thus the effects of pathogens on a given society are dependent to some degree on the human ecology of the society involved. This suggests that, in the face of a nosocomial pathogen such as SARS, social ingenuity may offset any lack of technical ingenuity and infrastructure.

Effect on International Health Governance

Before the emergence of SARS, international health regimes (as governed by the International Health Regulations) were badly dated, for two reasons. First, since their inception in 1951, the IHR had not been revised adequately in the face of other emerging novel pathogens. The member states of the WHO had last formally revised the IHR in 1969. Yet since 1970 humanity has witnessed the emergence of more than 30 previously unknown pathogens, and none of those were covered by the IHR in 2003, when they only required member states to report the incidence of smallpox, cholera, plague, and yellow fever. Further, under the provisions of the IHR the reporting of pathogen-induced morbidity and mortality remained the exclusive domain of sovereign member states. Countries have long sought to suppress the flow of information regarding endogenous epidemics, because the emergence of contagion typically generates significant negative effects on the economy and society of infected polities.[46] Thus, states have had significant material incentives to refrain from issuing timely and accurate reports on domestic epidemics to the global community. Beijing's early attempts to suppress the flow of information to the WHO and the insistence by Canadian officials that the WHO's travel advisories were erroneous both reflect this historical pattern of tension between sovereign member states and the WHO.

Nonetheless, some positive changes have taken place in the international health governance regime since the 1970s as a result of technological advances, the rise of new and reemerging infectious diseases, and the increasing involvement of non-state actors in addressing global microbial threats.

The WHO was instrumental in building the Global Outbreak Alert and Response Network, which was effectively mobilized to deal with the SARS contagion. Developed in 1997 and formalized in 2000, the GOARN is a network of approximately 120 partner networks engaged in pathogen detection, surveillance, and response. "During the response to SARS," the physician David Heynmann observed, "GOARN electronically linked some of the world's best laboratory scientists, clinicians, and epidemiologists in virtual networks that rapidly created and disseminated knowledge about the causative agent, mode of transmission, and other epidemiological features of SARS."[47]

During the World Health Assembly meetings of May 2003, member states of the World Health Organization stipulated that the organization should redouble its efforts to garner and analyze data from non-state actors. Specifically, the WHA requested that the Director-General of the WHO "take into account reports from sources other than official notification."[48] The new ability of non-state actors to communicate data directly to the WHO would seem to have broken the sovereign state's historical monopoly regarding the reporting of public health information, but this is only possible in those societies with sufficient telecommunications infrastructure.

In 1995, the WHO sought to revise the IHR so that the WHO could be allowed to use information from non-governmental organizations for epidemiological surveillance of infectious disease outbreaks.[49] Revisions to the IRH were finally completed in 2005, and member states must now immediately report the following pathogens to WHO: SARS coronavirus, novel strains of human influenza, smallpox, and polio. Adopted by the World Health Assembly in May 2005, the revised regime entered into force globally on June 15, 2007. The new regulations clarify the WHO's authority to recommend strategies of containment to member states, including various restrictions (such as quarantine) at ports, airports, and terrestrial borders and on means of international transportation.[50] This successful revision of the IHR, directly induced by the SARS scare, put an end to a decade of dithering by member states. Thus, SARS changed the calculus of the material interests of member states to reflect the threat that disease posed to their material interests, resulting in rapid innovation and change of the existing regime.

However, Fidler's arguments that we are now witness to a transformative or "post-Westphalian order that effectively limits the sovereign state's ability to compromise processes of global health governance under the auspices of international organizations (e.g., the WHO) are rather overstated. While the SARS epidemic appeared to have increased the power and authority of the WHO, the shift in power from sovereign states to the international organization was largely ephemeral. The sovereign state remains very capable of obfuscation through the non-reporting of disease data, and through other means of thwarting international efforts to address the spread of contagion. One need only look at the history of obfuscation and denial by political leaders in sub-Saharan Africa (Thabo Mbeki of South Africa and Robert Mugabe of Zimbabwe in particular) in the context of the HIV/AIDS pandemic to observe such obstruction.[51]

Theoretical Ramifications

The SARS epidemic exhibited emergent properties in that it featured a novel zoonotic pathogen (the SARS coronavirus) that jumped across animal reservoirs into the densely packed populations of southern China, whereupon it became endogenized in the human ecology of the region. It was then distributed via air travel throughout Southeast Asia, and from there to Canada. Finally, it appears that SARS was transmitted in nosocomial fashion, such that it thrived in the highly contained buildings of the developed world. Again, the epidemic that emerged was unanticipated and substantially greater than what would have been predicted by its constituent parts. Thus, globalization aided and abetted the emergence of the SARS epidemic. The psychological impacts of the contagion (fear, anxiety, stress) were greatly augmented by the actions of the global media, and by advances in telecommunications technology (such as the Internet and cell phones). However, on a positive note, such technological advances were also responsible for circumventing the suppression of data from China, thereby alerting the world to the mounting crisis.

Ultimately, it was not the global sharing of norms that led to the containment of SARS; rather, it was the sovereign state's concern for its material (primarily economic) interests that impelled states to take action to control SARS. In this case republican Realist theory provides a theoretical framework that explains the behavior of countries, particularly the desire to obscure the extent of the problem to the global community, and to initially resist the recommendations of international institutions (i.e. the WHO), even though such resistance may prove counterproductive and irrational over the longer term. Furthermore, the SARS epidemic reinforces the functional efficacy of the contagionist model and the postulates of the Florentine school, as pathogen containment was instituted by sovereign states through mechanisms of quarantine.

The outbreak of SARS is a good example of an "exogenous shock," emanating as it did from reservoirs in the natural world. It has undermined the Galenic mythology (still prevalent) that infectious disease is primarily a concern solely for the developing countries, with their limited levels of endogenous state capacity. Conversely, the SARS epidemic illustrates a central axiom of microbiology: that microbes will continue to evolve to colonize all available ecological niches, notwithstanding the wealth of a given society.[52] Therefore, as a result of the SARS contagion, developed countries realized that they too were vulnerable to the proliferation of debilitating and lethal pathogens.

One would logically expect that epistemic communities played a central role in proactively generating effective international regimes to deal with pathogens such as SARS, in that microbiologists effectively communicated their concerns to decision makers who then modified existing political regimes to deal with forthcoming epidemics. Unfortunately, such a proactive model is not borne out by the evidence, as the provisions of the IHR were not sufficiently revised to deal with emerging pathogens before the epidemic. At the domestic level, the influence of epistemic communities was similarly limited: in both the Chinese and Canadian examples, calls by scientists for greater investment in public health infrastructure were consistently ignored by political elites. Indeed, it is evident that domestic partisan politics resulted in significant erosion of Ontario's public health infrastructure, human capital, and funding base before the arrival of the SARS contagion.[53] Thus, domestic politics trumps the influence of epistemic communities in preparation for disease threats, perception of threat, and the efficacy of response to threat. In sum, given the limited influence of the public health community, countries typically exhibit reactive and not proactive stances regarding the surveillance and the control of infectious diseases.

Conclusions

By inflicting significant socio-economic costs on affected states, the SARS epidemic exposed the vulnerability of existing governance structures, reshaped the beliefs, norms, motivations, and preferences of individuals who weathered the crisis, and ultimately led to macro-level changes in domestic political governance, while enhancing the dynamics of regional health cooperation among the Pacific Rim countries. However, SARS-induced effects on the international system, and the relations of power between sovereign states and international organizations, were largely ephemeral. In this domain, the greatest effect of SARS was that it functioned as a catalyst to accelerate revision of the International Health Regulations and to get the list of reportable diseases updated.

SARS posed a significant material threat to the prosperity, effective governance, and security of affected states (China, Hong Kong, Canada, and Singapore in particular). Furthermore, SARS generated significant changes in public health governance within such affected states (particularly in Canada and China), leading to the formation of new institutions.

Conversely, and contrary to Fidler's assertions, the epidemic does not seem to have generated significantly increased compliance of sovereign states with international health regimes. Nor has the World Health Organization used the expanded powers it manifested during the SARS crisis, though arguably it could employ such strategies again to contain the burgeoning HIV/AIDS pandemic.

Why was the response to SARS so different from the relatively apathetic international reaction to HIV/AIDS, malaria, and tuberculosis? The SARS epidemic exhibited several factors that led to the temporary empowerment of the WHO: the emergence of a novel virus, coupled with seemingly high levels of virulence and transmissibility, generating high levels of uncertainty and fear. Further, the SARS epidemic was an exogenous shock that affected the material interests of global political and economic elites, and it presented an immediate socioeconomic crisis for decision makers to address at the national, regional, and international levels.

The case of SARS also illustrates the paradoxical role of modern technology in the face of novel outbreaks of contagion. Specifically, technology exhibited positive effects in the containment of SARS: cell phones and text messaging were used to transmit warnings from within China, facilitated the networked response of the WHO through the GOARN, and assisted in the accurate diagnosis of the pathogen. However, the rapid spread of the virus was accomplished through jet airplane technologies, nosocomial transmission was facilitated by modern hospital environments, and the global media played a significant role in generating anxiety and fear throughout the world.

Today, efforts to provide public goods such as improved global pathogen-surveillance systems and pathogen-containment regimes are the product of two central factors, namely fear and the attendant threat to the material interests of sovereign states (and global elites) generated by contagion. A significant amount of leadership to provide such public goods in the domain of public health has in fact been provided by hegemonic pressure from the United States, with the assistance of many other developed countries (and non-governmental organizations), in order to shore up surveillance and containment capacity within developing countries. This issue of regional and national capacity will continue to affect the dynamics of global health governance.[54]

7

War as a "Disease Amplifier"

Previous works have addressed the idea that infectious disease may manifest in epidemic or pandemic form through processes of amplification through ecological change.[1] Despite their analytical shortcomings, Galenic perspectives which specify that chronic poverty and the inequitable distribution of resources function as the principal (if not sole) variable involved in the spread of contagion are currently in vogue.[2] Poverty certainly does serve as an amplifier of pathogenic infection, however, it is not alone in this function as other variables, including ecological change, trade, migration, natural disasters,[3] and war may also serve as disease amplifiers. This chapter is primarily concerned with the effects of war (both inter-state and intra-state) on the emergence and proliferation of infectious disease. In it I argue that the processes of inter-state war and civil conflict create conditions directly conducive to the emergence, proliferation, and mutation of pathogens among both combatant and civilian populations. Thus war also functions as a "disease amplifier."

Of the various factors that "amplify" disease, this particular relationship is doubtless the least understood, and it requires the development of a robust theoretical construct of probable paths of causality. The intellectual soil has not remained utterly fallow, as historians have noted this relationship for centuries, and yet such issues remain relatively unexplored within the domain of political science. This chapter explores both historical sources, and the current available empirical data, in order to develop and refine a series of testable hypotheses to inform future work in this neglected area. To empirically establish this relationship I analyze previously unpublished data from the German and Austrian archives regarding the effects of World War I on disease-induced morbidity and mortality.

The causal relationship between conflict and infectious disease is rather complex, often exhibiting both emergent properties and non-linearities. The balance of the evidence presented herein suggests that war has historically functioned as a central catalyst in the propagation of infectious diseases. Conflict spreads contagion between (and within) factions of combatants, and then from the warring parties to the civilian populations that they come into contact with, both during and after the martial engagements in question. A second question, regarding causality, deals with the issue of whether infectious disease can generate conflict within societies, or between sovereign states. There is considerable weight to the proposition that war acts to amplify disease, but there is little current empirical evidence to support the hypothesis that disease fosters war between sovereign states.

Let us engage the first proposition, namely that war functions as a catalytic agent that facilitates the "emergence" of epidemic disease in a given polity or population. What do we then mean by "war" and "conflict"? For the most part the terms are used interchangeably to denote processes of armed aggression between two collectivities or factions of combatants.[4] This may manifest in war between two sovereign states (such as France and Germany) or in intra-state conflicts such as civil wars. The processes of conflict often generate the sufficient (although not necessary) conditions for the widespread diffusion of pathogens across the proximate region of conflict, and to those distal regions affected by demobilization. Thus, contagion might be passed from one force to another, and thereafter spread among the civilian populations through which the soldiers passed on their way home. At that point demobilized forces will then inadvertently spread pathogens within their own communities.

Critics

But what of the post-modernists who reject *a priori* any relationship between war and disease? The historian of science Roger Cooter argues that we must focus exclusively on the discourse and socio-historical "construction" of the partnership between war and disease, and ultimately he dismisses the concept of an empirical relationship between the two variables as pure fabrication, as a socially constructed discourse. He implores us to "concentrate on the different socio-political and professionalizing contexts within which the 'fatal partnership' between war and disease was fashioned, and eventually deposed, in epidemiology."[5]

Such extreme positions ring hollow, as there is no empirical epidemiological basis to Cooter's assertions. The data presented herein suggest the exact opposite: that an empirical relationship does very much exist, imperfect as the data may be. By denying the relationship between war and disease, post-modern scholars deliberately perpetuate ignorance regarding the relations between such variables, and thereby prevent any meaningful discussion of (and thereby impede the resolution of) these issues. Such obfuscation and denial, in the pursuit of ideology, paradoxically leads to greater harm for all over the long term, particularly the weak and disenfranchised.

Although analyses of the relationship between conflict and disease are novel in the domain of political science, the public health, medical, and historical communities have documented such issues for centuries. In the domain of public health, the epidemiologist Steve Morse has characterized war as a significant historical factor associated with the spread of infectious disease.[6] The epidemiologist William Foege concurs in his analysis of war's proximate and distal effects on population health. Foege argues that "organized violence, as seen in small or large conflicts, has direct and indirect effects on health as it leads to famines, epidemics, social dislocations, and the disruption of public health programs in general."[7] The medical historians Richard Garfield and Alfred Neugut agree, holding that social disruptions associated with the practices of war correlate with increases in the mortality rate among civilian populations. Such practices include "war-induced material deprivations (especially malnutrition), crowding, the breakdown of normal sanitary systems, and shortages of medical care. More casualties may be caused after wars than during wars."[8] The historian of medicine Hans Zinsser also understood this relationship between conflict and pestilence:

... war is ... 75 percent an engineering and sanitary problem, and a little less than 25 percent a military one. Other things being approximately equal, that army will win which has the best engineering and sanitary services. The wise general will do what the engineers and sanitary officers let him. The only reason why this is not entirely apparent in wars is because the military minds on both sides are too superb to notice that both armies are simultaneously immobilized by the same diseases.[9]

Theoretical Mechanisms

In this chapter I address the mechanisms by which warfare (either between sovereign states, or between factions within them) magnifies the distribution, and often the lethality, of epidemic disease. In 2000, Foege noted this lacuna in the modern literature, stating that "the impact of conflict on infectious diseases in the civilian population remains significant but insufficiently studied."[10] Here I hope to present some remedy to this problem, and to provoke further inquiries.

The medical geographers Matthew Smallman-Raynor and Andrew Cliff argue that conflict contributes to the proliferation of epidemic disease through a variety of biological and social interactions resulting from the ecology of war[11]:

... mobilization heightened mixing of both military and civil populations, thereby increasing the likelihood of disease transmission. Frequently, military personnel were drawn from a variety of epidemiological backgrounds, they were assembled and deployed in environments to which they were not acclimatized, and they carried infections for which the civil inhabitants of the war zones had little or no acquired immunity. For all involved resistance was further compromised by the mental and physical stress, trauma, nutritional deprivation and exposure to the elements. Insanitary conditions, enforced population concentration and crowding, a lack of medical provision, and the collapse of the conventional rules of social behaviour further compounded the epidemiological unhealthiness of war.[12]

By what mechanisms does war contribute to the emergence, proliferation, and increased lethality of pathogens? Processes of conflict (both intra-state or inter-state) often target, disrupt, and/or destroy public health infrastructure and medical facilities of those affected regions and/or countries, limiting the civil population's access to adequate health care and medicines. During war, civilian populations have a rational proclivity to flee zones of conflict, whereupon they may venture into novel regions occupied by certain endemic pathogens to which they may have little or no prior immunity. Conflict may induce widespread famine, or may otherwise dramatically increase the costs of available foodstuffs, both of which result in chronic and acute malnutrition that increases the host's susceptibility to pathogenic infection. Refugee populations exhibiting immunosuppression due to malnutrition (and psychological stress) may therefore be further victimized through increased levels of pathogenic infection. Further, with their mobility, malnourishment, lack of adequate shelter, and limited access to sufficient medical care, refugees are highly vulnerable to pathogenic colonization.[13] And warfare is historically associated with a breakdown in social norms, which typically manifests in an increased incidence of sexually transmitted diseases.

The virologist Paul Ewald has also noted the empirical association between warfare and infectious disease, and concurs with the argument that epidemics may exhibit war-induced "emergent properties." "Although the association between disease and warfare has long been recognized," Ewald writes, "it has been attributed solely to increased spread of pathogens and increased vulnerability of hosts. The possible effects of war on the evolution of pathogen characteristics has long been overlooked."[14] Ewald argues that the processes of conflict actually force the pathogens within the human host population to develop novel genetic attributes.

Historical Context

In 1916, the German medical historian Friedrich Prinzing argued that warfare was a proximate and direct cause of pathogenic infection, not only of military forces, but of civilian populations too.[15] The historian Paul Slack notes that historical archives are replete with accounts of epidemic diseases that afflicted and/or were distributed by military forces,[16] although the precise etiology of these pestilences remains indeterminate, hindered by the lack of diagnostic capacity in earlier eras. The historian J. N. Hays argued that military forces function as exceptionally effective conduits (vectors) of pathogenic dissemination, not only to other combatants but also to civil populations:

[As vectors] the armies of late medieval and early modern Europe afforded nearly ideal conditions: they contained large masses of unwashed and ill-nourished people living an undisciplined life in which they foraged over the countryside and lived in close proximity to others. And not only did armies propagate typhus; warfare disrupted whatever public health measures might be attempted. Not only did (the military) practice direct violence . . . it remained basically unwashed, itinerant, and promiscuous, a powerful agent for the diffusion of disease. And its enhanced destructive powers made it all the more likely that its incursions could completely break down the fabric of a community it attacked, including whatever provisions for health and sanitation existed.[17]

Let us examine the historical record in order to construct testable hypotheses regarding the diachronic relationship between conflict and contagion. Given that pathogens interact with the human ecology in different manners, particularly in the context of violent conflict, we conduct this inquiry by examining the role of individual pathogens.

Typhus

The first of the recorded "war pestilences" was the "plague" of Athens[18] (430–425 BC), which arose in Piraeus during the second year of the Peloponnesian War, shortly after the Peloponnesian invasion. According to Thucydides, trade and the conditions of war—particularly the flows of war refugees who were driven into Athens (and the resulting exceptional population densities)—played pivotal roles in the rise of the epidemic.[19] Ergo, a contributing factor to the outbreak of contagion would seem to be massive population movements from rural to urban centers (in this case Athens), generating exceptional population densities that were epidemiologically permissive to the pathogenic colonization of the population. Zinsser concurs, and attributes the pathogen's emergence directly to the conditions associated with the ongoing conflict, such as dense military encampments and the movement of materiel from Africa.[20] Moreover, once the contagion was established within Athens, the Athenian military apparently served as an efficient vector for diffusion of the pathogen, even as it was simultaneously depleted by the disease. Zinsser notes that "the pestilence followed the Athenian fleet, which was attacking the Peloponnesian coast, and prevented the carrying out of the objectives for which the expedition had been organized."[21]

Notwithstanding the nascent body of genetic evidence that typhus visited Greece during the Peloponnesian War, it appears to have burned itself out or gone into hibernation, as it was some time before it revisited European societies. Hays argues that the next confirmed appearance of typhus on European soil (after the Peloponnesian War) occurred in 1489–90, during (and perhaps resulting from) the Spanish conflict with the Moors over the possession of Granada.[22] The historian William McNeill concurs with the temporal frame of typhus' introduction into European societies (circa 1490), but he offers a different explanation of the pathogen's geographic origins. Typhus, he writes, "made its debut on European soil in 1490, when it was brought to Spain by soldiers who had been fighting in Cyprus. Thence it came into Italy with the wars between Spaniards and French for dominion over that peninsula. Typhus achieved a new notoriety in 1526 when a French army besieging Naples was compelled to withdraw in disarray due to the ravages of the disease."[23] From this point on, typhus became endogenized within the European human ecology, and its proliferation became associated with violent conflict.

Persistent conflicts between European forces and the Ottoman Empire facilitated the spread of typhus throughout Europe during the 1500s.

Prinzing argues that in the latter years of the fifteenth century Hungary was destabilized by typhus, which had been brought to that country as a result of the protracted conflict with the Ottoman Empire:

... hitherto prosperous Hungary, by endless wars with Turkey ... was brought to the very edge of ruin.... the utter lack of sanitation, increased the baneful effects of camp life. Dirt and refuse accumulated in heaps, vermin multiplied so rapidly that it was impossible to get rid of them, corpses were inadequately buried, while enormous numbers of flies and gnats molested the soldiers and did a great deal toward spreading infectious diseases. The hospitals were in a pitiable condition ... [and] the soldiers ... gave themselves over to a most dissolute life.... A large part of the German troops never once faced the enemy, for the reason that they succumbed beforehand to "Hungarian disease" (i.e. typhus), which killed more of them than the swords of the Turks. Hence Hungary was called at that time the "Cemetery of the Germans."[24]

The war-induced diffusion of typhus facilitated the first pan-European epidemic of the pestilence in 1566, as the disease became ubiquitous during the war between Maximilian II and the Turks, then spread into western lands. "After the dispersion of the (Habsburg) army," Prinzing writes, "the discharged soldiers carried the disease in all directions. Vienna was hit very hard.... The returning Italians brought the disease first to Carinthia ... and then to Italy. In the same way it was carried to Bohemia, Germany, Burgundy, Belgium, and Spain."[25]

In the seventeenth century the spread of typhus was also greatly facilitated by the horrid conditions of the Thirty Years' War (1618–1648), by troop movements, and by the widespread conflict-induced famine that eroded the immunological vigor of affected populations. "In the history of this calamitous war," the Prussian historian Friedrich Seitz wrote, "we see typhus fever like a malignant specter hovering over the armies wherever they go, in their camps, on their marches, and in their permanent quarters, and preparing an inglorious end for thousands of valiant warriors. Its ravages among the non-belligerent population in town and country caused the inhabitants of many provinces to remember with hatred and loathing the departed soldiers...."[26] Prinzing concurs: "... epidemics of dysentery, typhus fever, and bubonic plague followed at the heels of armies (and thus) were borne from place to place, ... the great depopulation of Germany during the Thirty Years' War was chiefly caused by epidemics of typhus fever and bubonic plague."[27] Typhus would also seem to have contributed to the destruction of French forces during Napoleon's withdrawal of the Grand Armée from Russia in

1812.[28] Indeed, typhus was one of the numerous infections that beset Napoleon's forces as they marched toward Moscow from their bases in Central Europe during the summer of 1811:

After the battle of Smolensk (August 14–18, 1811) ... typhus fever and other diseases ... continued to spread throughout the army. The most common disease even in Moscow was typhus fever. ... When Napoleon's army withdrew from the city it left behind several thousand typhus fever patients, almost all of whom died. ... The horrors of the return march are well known. ... The number of sick soldiers was enormous, and typhus fever raged more and more extensively. In pursuing the French army the Russians also suffered severely from diseases. ... between October 20 and December 14, 1812, they lost 61,964 men, most of whom died of "nerve fever" (typhus fever).[29]

Thus, both the Napoleonic and the Russian army served as primary vectors of contagion, and their movements subsequently generated epidemic typhus in the cities that lay in the path of the combatants (e.g., Vilnius, Warsaw, and St. Petersburg). According to H. A. Goden, a physician in the French forces, the military hospitals (lazarets) of the time also functioned as effective nodes of pestilential diffusion in the wake of the dispersing Grand Armée.[30] The Prussian physician Heinrich Haser corroborates this description of disbanded troops, and their military hospitals, serving as highly effective vectors of transmission throughout Central Europe:

French soldiers returning from Russia ... spread the contagion of various diseases over a large part of Central Europe. Almost naked, or clothed in ... rags, without shoes ... and their frozen limbs covered with festering sores, they marched through Poland and Germany. Typhus fever and other diseases ... marked their course. The inhabitants of the country were forced to house the sick; but teamsters also conveyed the infection to villages which the soldiers did not visit. The disease raged most furiously in the hospitals.[31]

The contagion also appears to have visited the Americas, and it became particularly pernicious during the hostilities associated with the American Revolutionary War (1775–1783). The US medical historian Ted Woodward noted that during the American Revolution typhus infected, and debilitated, approximately one-third of the New York Army of General Nathaniel Greene in 1776, immediately before a confrontation with British forces.[32]

Modern skeptics may certainly argue that much of this argument is based on anecdotal evidence, or may otherwise question the validity of such accounts. However, the German medical archives of World War I, as prepared by German military physicians, provide us with solid empirical data to support the hypothesis that conflict can act as a mechanism of transmission of epidemic typhus. In this case the onset of the war initiated a massive outbreak of typhus among the German armed forces in the months immediately after the initiation of hostilities. (See figure 7.1.)

During the years 1916–1918, medical innovations resulted in the reduction of incidence and typhus-induced mortality. Despite the increasing capacity of the Germans to control the spread of typhus, it spread inexorably eastward in the months that followed the formal cessation of hostilities in November 1918. Consequently, the pestilence infected millions throughout Eastern Europe and Russia, with estimated civilian and military mortality exceeding 100,000. The military physician Brown notes that during this period approximately one-third of physicians in the Soviet Red Army contracted typhus, and 20 percent of those perished of the disease.[33] This dynamic of post-conflict diffusion followed the pattern of earlier epidemics as demobilizing forces again served as agents that transmitted the louse vector, and therefore *Rickettsia*, throughout a vast area.

During World War II the incidence of typhus in European forces declined dramatically as military units made hygiene a priority. However, that war temporally coincided with epidemic outbreaks in those geographic regions where public health capacity was greatly diminished as a result of the hostilities. Specifically, the physician Bavaro notes that "during and immediately after the war hundreds of thousands of cases of typhus, with up to 10 percent mortality rates, appeared in civilian populations in Egypt, French North Africa, Naples, Germany, Japan, and Korea."[34] The manifestations of the illness, and the impact on both military and civilian populations were far more pronounced in the Pacific theater of operations. "In that preantibiotic era, the disease sometimes caused more casualties than actual combat, with mortality rates exceeding 27 percent. There were more than 20,000 cases among Japanese forces and 16,000 cases among Allied troops, including more than 7,300 cases and 331 deaths among US troops."[35] The last major recorded outbreak of conflict-induced typhus occurred during the Korean War. Although typhus was largely contained within the military populations of the UN alliance, the material deprivation and destruction of public health infrastructure resulting from the war spawned an outbreak of typhus that resulted in approximately 32,000 cases and 6,000 deaths among South Korean military and civilian populations.[36]

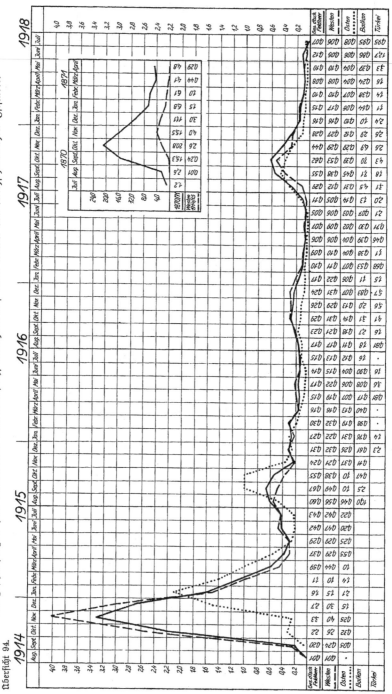

Figure 7.1
Typhus morbidity, German armed forces, 1914–1918. Source: *Sanitätsbericht über das deutsche heer im Weltkriege 1914/1918,* volume 3 (Mittler & Sohn, 1934).

Smallpox

Variola established itself in East Asia after the Chinese General Ma-Yuan employed military forces to suppress a Wuling revolt in Hunan province in the years 48–49 AD. The historian Donald Hopkins writes:

The general led his army into a district where an epidemic was in progress. The result was that more than half of the Chinese expeditionary force, including General Ma-Yuan, succumbed to the disease. The remnants of Ma-Yuan's army returned home with their prisoners, bringing "captives pox," or "barbarian pox" into China.[37]

The Antonine Plague that ravaged the Roman Empire in 166–168 AD exhibited symptoms that bore a close resemblance to smallpox. According to Prinzing, the contagion was the result of military vectors transporting the pathogen from the Levant back to the Empire. Specifically, General Avidius Cassius (preceding Verus) was deployed to Syria in order to suppress rebellious local factions, and *Variola* appeared during the capture of Seleucia. From that point "it was borne by the troops back to Rome, where, after the triumphal procession of 166, it spread far and wide. . . . The plague spread from Italy to Gaul, to the very banks of the Rhine, and a large part of the province was significantly depopulated—decayed and deserted villages were found everywhere."[38]

Variola appears to have been firmly established in the Arab world around 622 AD, and the vectors and conditions associated with warfare accelerated the spread of the pathogen throughout that region. "After Alexandria," Hopkins writes, "the Arab armies swept across western Asia, North Africa, and conquered Spain before they were stopped at Constantinople in 717, and at Poitiers, France, in 732. Smallpox went with them, into Syria, Palestine, Sicily, Mauritania, Spain, and France."[39] Furthermore, the Crusades in the twelfth and thirteenth centuries apparently reintroduced and facilitated the spread of *Variola* across European societies. "Pox houses" became ubiquitous along the paths trod by Crusaders returning from the Levant to England via Germany.[40]

In later years, smallpox influenced the outcome of the conflict between the nascent United States and the Dominion of Canada. During the American Revolutionary War, the contagion played a role in debilitating the US Army. Benedict Arnold led a massive force of colonial troops against the British colony, and after the capture of Montreal the contagion entered the ranks of the American forces en route to Quebec City. American forces buried their dead in mass graves as they retreated in disorder.[41] "Of the 10,000 troops in the attack, 5,500 developed smallpox. There were not enough tents to shelter even the desperately sick men. The moans of the sick and dying could be heard everywhere. Pits were opened as common graves and filled day after day with corpses as the men died like flies."[42] Thomas Jefferson later commented that *Variola* had been "sent into our army designedly by the (British) commanding officer in Quebec," although such claims have never been empirically verified.[43] According to Oldstone's analysis, approximately 55 percent of US forces in this particular campaign developed smallpox and were killed, nullifying the United States' capacity to project military power within this theatre and allowing the continuation of British rule within North America.[44] Fenn notes that after the disastrous campaign against Quebec the demobilizing US forces were highly effective vectors for the spread of the contagion throughout New York, Connecticut, and Pennsylvania.[45]

Prinzing argued that the Franco-Prussian War operated as the central epidemiological catalyst that generated the devastating smallpox epidemic of 1870–71. This contagion was the scourge of both Prussia's and France's populations (military and civilian) and resulted in approximately 300,000 fatalities.[46] The French physician Andre Laveran noted that this particular epidemic of smallpox began in France and circulated throughout French military forces before their deployment against Prussia.[47] Prinzing speculated that field soldiers in general and French prisoners of war in particular served as agents of pathogenic transmission to Prussian populations. In particular, the prisoner-of-war camps in Prussia functioned as nodes in a network of pathogenic distribution that facilitated the spread of smallpox to the Prussian civilian population. The medical historian James Rolleston concurs, stating that "the epidemic would seem to have originated in France, but then mutated into a haemorrhagic form as it was spread by French troop vectors into the states of Prussia and its allies."[48] This explosion of smallpox mortality temporally coincided with the onset of hostilities, whereupon the mortality associated with the pathogen increased by an order of magnitude. (See figure 7.2.) Smallpox subsequently continued its pattern of diffusion into the civilian population, persisting well beyond the formal cessation of hostilities in 1871. The mortality induced by the war-pestilence reached its zenith in 1872, and thereafter declined in equally dramatic fashion.

The historian Richard Evans observed that soldiers returning to Hamburg from the Franco-Prussian war served as effective conduits of

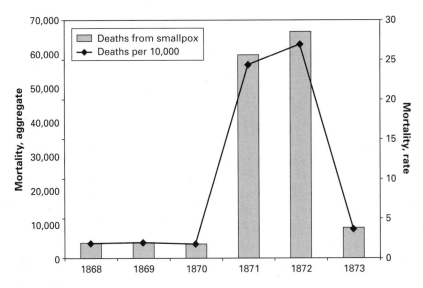

Figure 7.2
Prussian mortality from smallpox, 1868–1873.

transmission, resulting in the deaths of 4,043 residents of Hamburg by *Variola* in 1871. Such mortality generated a mortality rate of "15.4 per 1000, which made the smallpox outbreak of 1871 the greatest of all epidemics in nineteenth-century Hamburg. . . . 9,055 victims were hospitalized, of whom 908 died. If this ratio of deaths to cases held good for those not treated in hospital, then there may have been 40,000 cases. . . . 29 percent of all deaths in Hamburg in 1871 were caused by smallpox."[49]

Smallman-Raynor and Cliff argue that Prinzing was indeed correct in his assertions that the geographical diffusion of smallpox during the Franco-Prussian War was very much facilitated by the network of prisoner-of-war camps. In conducting their analysis, Smallman-Raynor and Cliff employ data originally collected by the Prussian medical statistician Albert Guttstadt.[50] The analysis involved geospatial multivariate regression, in order to determine that the war directly contributed to the proliferation of smallpox among the Prussian military and civilian populations. Smallman-Raynor and Cliff argue that smallpox "spread through the civil system of urban centres as a mixed diffusion process with a dominant hierarchical component. Contrary to expectation, however, this process . . . was determined by the system of POW camps that had developed around the urban system during the course of the war."[51] They conclude that "the exigencies of war may result in a fundamental reconfiguration of epidemic diffusion processes in civil settlement systems."[52]

Plague (*Yersinia pestis*)

Hans Zinsser argued that pathogenic co-infectivity during a protracted conflict exhibited enormous complexity and variation over time. He argued that it is possible to divide the biological history of the Thirty Years' War (1618–1648) into two distinct epidemiological periods, with typhus reigning from 1618 to 1630. Thereafter, from 1630 to 1648, bubonic plague rose to become the premier scourge of those countries party to the conflict. On an epidemiological level this succession of contagion makes sense as those exposed to typhus would either have been killed, or thereafter acquired some immunity to the pathogen, clearing the way for the ascension of a pathogen to which they had little or no prior immunity (*Yersinia pestis*). However, during this epic era of societal chaos and inter-state war, various and diverse pathogens; dysentery, typhoid fever, smallpox, and scarlet fever, all interacted with typhus and plague.

Once again soldiers proved to be highly efficient vectors of pathogenic distribution. After the return of bubonic plague in 1630, it "traveled with the rapidly moving armies, remaining behind when the soldiers departed, and spreading from innumerable foci into the surrounding country."[53] It is noteworthy that even into the nineteenth century, the disease continued to be problematic for military forces, and the conduct of martial campaigns. August Hirsch observed that the conflict between Russian and Turkish forces in Wallachia in 1828–29 generated the last significant outbreak of Bubonic Plague in the European theatre.[54]

Thereafter, the incidence of plague in the European population diminished markedly as sanitary measures improved. Yet *Yersinia pestis* would continue to afflict societies in East Asia for some time to come. Hays notes that the armed rebellion of 1855 in Yunnan province of China facilitated the spread of the pathogen throughout the entire region: "The great Muslim rebellion that began in 1855 resulted in nearly two decades of internal turmoil in Yunnan, in which plague epidemics coincided with military massacres, famine, and considerable emigration.... Troop movements and emigration may have spread plague to other areas of China."[55] This association between war and plague continued into the twentieth century as a significant outbreak of plague struck down thousands of Vietnamese citizens from 1966 to 1974, primarily as a result of the atrocious conditions associated with the war; including the destruction of health infrastructure, and breakdown of hygiene and sanitary measures.[56] Antibiotic prophylaxis has proved to be crucial to the containment of *Yersinia pestis*, yet the pathogen remains endemic at low levels throughout some regions of the world, including the American Southwest.

Cholera

The diffusion of *Vibrio* was also often associated with the movements of troops who carried it to vulnerable populations. Such conflict-induced epidemics were certainly not confined to European soil, as war proved to be the pivotal vector of the transmission of cholera from its reservoirs in South Asia (i.e. India) to Europe. Evans argues that one of the first of such transmissions occurred when, "the Marquess of Hastings fought a military campaign against the Marathas in 1817, losing 3,000 out of 10,000 troops to the disease in the process." From that point the contagion traveled via various routes, through other proximate military campaigns, until it reached England.[57] William McNeill concurs: "British troops fighting a series of campaigns along India's northern frontiers between 1816 and 1818 carried the cholera with them from their headquarters in Bengal, and communicated the disease to their Nepalese and Afghan enemies. Military movements connected with Russia's wars against Persia (1826–28) and Turkey (1828–29) . . . carried the cholera to the Baltic by 1831, whence it spread by ship to England."[58] Hirsch supports this line of argument as well, noting that the spread of cholera throughout Poland and the Baltic region during the 1830s was very much related to conflict, stating that the "military operations of the Russo-Polish War contributed materially to its diffusion."[59]

It was from this foothold in Eastern Europe that cholera began its inexorable march across the fertile and immunologically naive populations of Europe. Evans concurs that Russian military actions to thwart the Polish rebellion in 1831 created the pre-conditions, abetted by conflict-induced waves of Polish refugees, that allowed for the rapid spread of *Vibrio* to Central and ultimately Western Europe. Furthermore, he argues that the Crimean War also contributed to the pathogens diffusion throughout the Continent and Asia Minor: "In 1854 French troops embarking for Gallipoli and Varna at Marseilles and Toulon carried cholera with them and ensured that a major outbreak occurred when they finally reached the theatre of war in the Crimea."[60] Finally, the destabilization induced by the Austro-Prussian War of 1866 appeared to have contributed directly to the rise of epidemic cholera in Austria-Hungary, which induced approximately 165,000 deaths in that year.[61]

Few modern empirical studies have tested the empirical relationship between war, and vectors of pathogenic diffusion, in the domain of cholera. The most revealing (and methodologically sophisticated) medical-spatial regressions to date have been conducted by Smallman-Raynor and Cliff, who examined the dynamics of the diffusion of epidemic cholera in the Philippines during the Philippine-American War (1902–1904). They consequently determined that "the mass population movements associated with the war had the effect of speeding up the geographical propagation of cholera as compared with peace," although the fundamental geographical channels of disease spread remained in effect.[62]

Influenza

McNeill suggests, correctly, that the horrific conditions generated during the course of World War I, and contact between troops of disparate geographical origins, may have accelerated the evolution of a lethal and highly transmissible pandemic influenza that killed millions in 1918–19.[63] Oxford et al. concur that the influenza pandemic of 1918 was likely facilitated and indeed intensified by the conditions of the protracted war in Europe.[64] It does seem reasonable to argue that the epidemiologically malign conditions of the western front, notably the exceptional population densities associated with trench warfare, contributed to the evolution of increasingly lethal waves of the pandemic as it circled the world, with troop movements serving as vectors. Perhaps the best empirical argument to support the notion of the 1918 pandemic as exhibiting emergent properties deriving from World War I is proffered by the virologist Paul Ewald:

One of the best examples of an evolutionary increase in virulence is the influenza pandemic of 1918. The environmental conditions associated with the trench warfare of World War I could hardly have been more favorable for the evolution of increased virulence of airborne pathogens like influenza. Soldiers in the trenches were grouped so closely that even immobile infecteds could transmit pathogens. The sick individuals were generally moved between a succession of crowded rooms by a succession of crowded vehicles. The severely sick and badly wounded were then sent within a few hours by trucks to one or more evacuation hospitals and then eventually by railcars to base hospitals. Additional new susceptibles would be transported to the trenches to take the place of ill people who had been removed. As the trenchmates infected by an already removed soldier became ill, the process continued. In the camps away from the trenches, the high densities of soldiers and transport of sick and susceptible soldiers may have contributed to increased virulence by a similar mechanism. The increased mortality in the trenches due to fighting or the other infectious diseases that typically accompanied such warfare should have, if anything, also favored a high level of virulence. If the conditions and activities at the western front were responsible for the enhanced virulence of the 1918 pandemic, the timing and spatial pattern of virulent disease should accord with virulence enhancement at the western front....[65]

The data presented by Alfred Crosby appear to support Ewald's hypothesis that the war, and the activities on the western front in particular, served as an amplifier of the contagion, accelerating its proliferation among susceptible hosts, and thereby increasing its lethality.[66] The only caveat to Ewald's argument is that, as I have argued above, the first manifestations of a highly lethal influenza may have actually appeared in Austria during the spring of 1917, reinforcing Oxford's hypothesis that the influenza emerged and evolved within the European theatre before its apparent emergence in highly lethal form in Kansas during the spring of 1918. Ewald's argument does help to explain how the lethality of the virus intensified in the horrid conditions of the western front, and was augmented in each of the three waves as it circled the world, propelled by the continual movements of troops serving as highly efficient vectors.

Tuberculosis

The "White Plague" has been the bane of human societies for millennia, and it continues to debilitate and kill millions per year, even in the era of antibiotics. The association of tuberculosis with conflict is an area that is rather unexplored, yet the association makes intuitive sense. Theoretically, soldiers under stress will experience weakened immune systems, and malnourishment will further compromise immunity. Significant population densities in military camps and trenches would certainly facilitate the communication of the pathogen between susceptible troops, and one would expect that the processes of war would increase the incidence of, and perhaps the mortality associated with tuberculosis. Again, the German medical records from World War I illustrate this

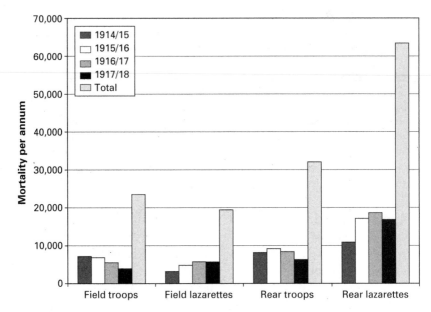

Figure 7.3
Tuberculosis mortality, German armed forces, 1914–1918. Source: *Sanitätsbericht über das deutsche heer im Weltkriege 1914/1918*, volume 3 (Mittler & Sohn, 1934).

relationship, and provide preliminary empirical evidence to support this association. (See figure 7.3.) One can certainly discern an increase in tuberculosis-induced mortality from 1914 until 1916, whereupon the mortality rate appears to plateau and thereafter decline somewhat toward the end of the war. This suggests that the onset of the war had a moderate effect on increasing both the incidence and the mortality associated with the pathogen in German forces.

A comparison of the German military data with the Austrian records of tuberculosis-induced civilian mortality in Vienna is expedient. The Austrian data provide us with a prewar baseline of 4,924 deaths in 1912, peaking at 9,650 deaths in 1917, and declining to 8,539 deaths in 1919. The data clearly indicate that the onset and progression of the war is directly associated with the dramatic increase in tuberculosis-induced mortality in Vienna. Furthermore, the epidemic of tuberculosis intensifies in the latter years of the war, and indeed this pattern persists into the postwar period. Another point to consider is that the increasing mortality associated with tuberculosis in 1919 may reflect the destructive effects of the 1918 influenza pandemic, which certainly weakened the lung tissues and immune systems of survivors, making them vulnerable to secondary bacterial infections of which tuberculosis would be a prime candidate. This further illustrates the complex interactivity and connectivity of pathogens in the context of the human ecology.

In more recent times, the attenuated conflict in Afghanistan between United States and newly resurgent Taliban forces has apparently amplified the incidence of tuberculosis in that country. The epidemiologists Ibrahim Khan and Ulrich Laaser argue that the war has directly contributed to the increasing incidence of the disease among the general population, with attendant increases in mortality.[67] Aside from generating the preconditions that facilitate pathogenic diffusion and colonization of hosts, the war has also impeded efforts by international organizations (e.g., the WHO), and non-governmental organizations (e.g., Medicins Sans Frontieres) to bring the contagion under control. Specifically, the diffuse conflict has impeded comprehensive epidemiological surveys of the population, such that only sporadic surveys are possible. It has also resulted in the erosion of the endogenous public health infrastructure, or prevented the establishment of such infrastructure in highly impoverished areas. Moreover, the nature of the conflict has impeded the delivery of effective medical treatment to those suffering from infection. This requires the consistent provision of medicines to those infected, who must in turn follow a prolonged regimen of treatment. Khan and Laaser elaborate:

War extremely reduces the chance of regular therapy among patients and limits access to regular health care in every conflict area.... Over one third of the country has no routine immunization program.... Dormant tuberculosis bacilli can spring back to life and cause illness when people are especially stressed, not adequately nourished, immunocompromised, or in close contact with the infection source. The circumstances in refugee camps are extremely poor and there is a high risk of infection and re-infection.[68]

Moreover, refugees also serve as conduits of infection to other proximate countries. In this particular case, it would appear that the war has exacerbated the prevalence of endemic tuberculosis, which is now spreading from its reservoir in Afghanistan through population movements (primarily civilians fleeing conflict) to neighboring Pakistan.[69] In this manner we see the interactivity between war and disease, with the former reinforcing the latter. In this sense then the global public bad of war clearly serves to exacerbate another public bad, the tuberculosis pandemic.

Malaria

The spread of malaria is related to many factors, including poverty, but it is also very much related to environmental change, specifically changes in land use, changes in water use (i.e., dams and irrigation) and transportation infrastructure that permitted the migration of the *plasmodium* through human vectors. It should not come as a surprise then that the conditions associated with conflict might contribute to epidemics of malaria in immunologically naive populations, and even to establish the disease in those geographic zones where it had not been previously endemic. Evidence of the latter comes from the highlands of Western Kenya, which were free of malaria for much of their recorded history. In this case, changes in land use and transportation infrastructure, such as the extension of the railroad from the coast in 1901, allowed for the gradual establishment of the plasmodium in the regional ecology. However, epidemic malaria was only first reported in the region in the second decade of the twentieth century. The epidemiologist Mark Malakooti and his co-workers conclude that troop demobilization after World War I was the premier factor in establishing malaria throughout that region: "The first reported epidemic was in 1918 to 1919 when local soldiers returned from Tanzania after World War I. Two epidemics were recorded in the 1920s and four in the 1930s. After the military camp in the area was disbanded in 1944, the local outbreaks ceased, but highland malaria continued to be a serious public health problem until the late 1950s. . . ."[70]

Dysentery (*Shigella*)

As was noted above, war is often characterized by interaction between various pathogens. Aside from the smallpox induced by conditions of the Franco-Prussian War, numerous other diseases were transmitted during the course of that campaign including dysentery which generated an extraordinary level of morbidity among the troops. "Of the German field-army," Prinzing writes, "38,975 men, all told, contracted dysentery (47.8 per 1,000 of the average number of troops under arms), and of these 2,405 died. Of the average number of French prisoners taken to Germany 41.7 percent contracted the disease. . . ."[71] McNeil concurs: ". . . in even the best-managed armies, disease was always a far more lethal factor than enemy action, even during active campaigns. In the Crimean War (1854–56), for example, ten times as many British soldiers died of dysentery as from all the Russian weapons put together. . . ."[72]

Data collected by the German medical services indicate that the incidence of dysentery (described as "Ruhr" in the German records) in the German forces increased dramatically as the war continued, peaking in 1918. This pattern of increase is consistent with the reports of poor nutrition and declining health infrastructure throughout the country. (See figure 7.4.)

Sexually Transmitted Diseases

Armies have also functioned as optimal vectors for the transmission of syphilis and other sexually transmitted diseases. The historical appearance of syphilitic infection in European populations closely followed on the heels of the Columbian "discovery" of the Americas. Indeed, Crosby posits that syphilis was imported to Europe by Iberian troops during the initial phases of the conquest of the Americas.[73] Anthropological evidence suggests that syphilis (*Treponema pallidum* or Treponema S), which is genetically similar to yaws (Treponema Y), was imported to Europe from the Americas by the Spaniards during and after 1492.[74] "The disease," Watts argues, "then mutated in their bodies . . . to become the *Treponema pallidum* which suddenly was so much in evidence among the French mercenary army which invaded Italy in 1494."[75] The virulence of the syphilis epidemics that swept Europe in the fifteenth and sixteenth centuries was of such magnitude that it suggests the bacterium was devastating a population that had acquired no prior immunity through exposure to the pathogen. In other words, European populations were apparently immunologically naive. War had a now familiar role to play in the subsequent diffusion of syphilis across the Continent. During the siege of Naples by the French armies of Charles VIII in 1494, the latter's troops bore the contagion of syphilis with them. "There the French army gave itself over to the most unbridled licentiousness, and the result was that [syphilis] spread rapidly in both the French and Italian armies. The disbanding of Charles's army caused the disease to spread far and wide in Europe."[76] McNeill concurs, arguing that syphilis made its first appearance in epidemic form during the long series of Franco-Italian conflicts in the period 1494–1559: "[Syphilis] broke out in epidemic fashion in the army that the French king, Charles VIII, led against Naples in 1494. When the French withdrew, King Charles thereupon discharged his soldiers, who thereupon spread the disease far and wide to all adjacent lands."[77] Thereafter, syphilis became an endemic pathogen that colonized European populations, its virulence declining through

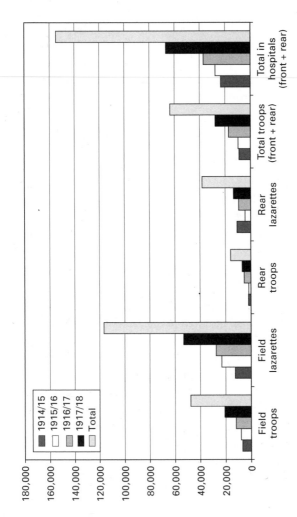

Figure 7.4
Dysentery morbidity, German armed forces, 1914–1918. Source: as for figure 3.2.

mutual pathogen-host adaptation. It persists to this day all over the world.

HIV

As of the time of writing (2008), two clades of the human immunodeficiency virus have become endogenized within the human ecology, with HIV-1 exhibiting global diffusion whereas HIV-2 has become widespread predominantly throughout western Africa. In their analysis of the distribution of HIV-1, Smallman-Raynor and Cliff determined that the distribution of the pathogen in Central and East Africa is highly correlated with the distribution of conflict, and with recruitment vectors in the region. Specifically, they argue that "both the spread of HIV 1 infection in the 1980s, and the subsequent development of AIDS to its 1990 spatial pattern, are shown to be significantly and positively correlated with ethnic patterns of recruitment into the Ugandan National Liberation Army (UNLA) after the overthrow of Idi Amin some ten years earlier in 1979." Their data suggest that both the "truck-town" hypothesis (according to which transportation vectors determine the distribution of the pathogen) and the "migrant labor" hypothesis (according to which the pathogen is diffused from urban centers of labor demand to rural areas that possess a supply of labor) are inaccurate in predicting the present pattern of pathogenic diffusion. Specifically, multivariate regressions that analyze the spatial distribution of the epidemic indicate that the Ugandan civil war of 1979–1985 is the greatest predictor of the distribution of the pathogen.[78]

A team of geneticists and demographers led by Philippe Lemey reconstructed the evolution of the HIV-2 epidemic from its established locus of origin in Guinea-Bissau. They found that the virus shifted from endemic to epidemic status in the period 1955–1970, which coincides with that country's war of independence from Portugal. Lemey et al. write:

Our demographic estimates suggest that an event enabled HIV-2 subtype A to switch to epidemic growth sometime around 1955–1970. An initiation of the epidemic at this time coincides with the time frame of the independence war (1963–1974) in Guinea-Bissau. . . . There is evidence that both sexual and blood-borne HIV-2 transmission markedly increased during this period. Epidemiological linkage of HIV-2 with Portugal, established during the presence of the colonial army, was recognized when the first reported cases of HIV-2 in Europe were Portuguese veterans who had served in the army during the independence war.[79]

According to the military analyst Lindy Heinecken, a significant proportion of African military forces exhibit HIV seroprevalence rates
ranging from 40 percent to 60 percent.[80] Although this estimate may be
elevated, there are few solid empirical data to refute it, as many states
have defined such data as classified. The political scientist Stefan Elbe
has written extensively on the role of soldiers as highly effective vectors
of HIV transmission, particularly in the context of sub-Saharan Africa.
He notes that soldiers are "of a sexually active age; they are highly
mobile and away from home for long periods of time; they often valorize
violent and risky behavior; they have greater opportunities for casual
sexual relations; and they may seek to relieve themselves from the stress
of combat through sexual activity."[81] Martin Schonteich concurs, but
further argues that armed conflict often leads to an increased frequency
of sexual coercion, often to the rape of civilians by military personnel.[82]
In this vein of inquiry, Elbe presents convincing evidence that "war-rape"
is increasingly used as deliberate weapon of war. He states that "the
deliberate transmission of HIV/AIDS has been used in Africa at a
minimum as a psychological weapon of war to induce further anxiety
among females in societies that have become war zones. Preliminary
evidence suggests that the HIV prevalence rate among rape survivors is
high. Two-thirds of a recent sample of 1,200 Rwandan genocide widows
tested positive for HIV."[83] Elbe continues: ". . . appropriations of HIV/
AIDS by armed forces in Africa reflect the virus's increasing significance
as a weapon of war. Combatants have sought to use the psychological
and lethal effects of HIV/AIDS to gain strategic advantage over their
opponents."[84] It is difficult to state definitively that this is a departure
from past practices, as soldiers infected by pathogens have engaged in
practices of sexual coercion and rape of civilians throughout recorded
history. The difference in this case is that such practices are apparently
being used in deliberate and strategic fashion to undermine the morale
and social cohesion of the enemy.

On Mortality from Co-Infection

As was noted above, one analytical problem is the issue of the co-
infection of troops and civilian populations by multiple pathogens. It is
certainly reasonable to assume that over the span of an attenuated conflict (such as the Thirty Years' War) that the forces and populations
involved experienced a succession of epidemics, often with multiple

sources of infection. World War I saw the infection of German and Austrian populations by influenza, which then opened the way for subsequent epidemics of pneumonia and tuberculosis. This makes any such strict accounting of influenza-induced mortality rather problematic, in that the secondary effects of the pandemic persisted for some time. This reinforces the position taken by the political scientist Hazem Ghobarah et al. that the public health costs of wars (and complex emergencies) are likely complex, attenuated, and difficult to estimate.

Disease-induced mortality data from the US Civil War provide us with some idea of the relative aggregate mortality from disease vs. battlefield injuries. The mortality statistics on Union troops compiled by US Surgeon-General Barnes in 1870–1888 are the best available data on causes of death during that conflict.[85] The data indicate that deaths from infectious diseases vastly exceeded battlefield deaths and deaths from wounds suffered in action. (See figure 7.5.) It is instructive to compare aggregate battlefield and wound-induced mortality (93,443) against deaths from infectious disease. The ratio of disease-induced mortality to battlefield/wound-induced mortality is a significant 1.9928:1, suggesting that disease was very much a security issue to American forces during this era. But such data were not disaggregated into mortality by specific pathogen,

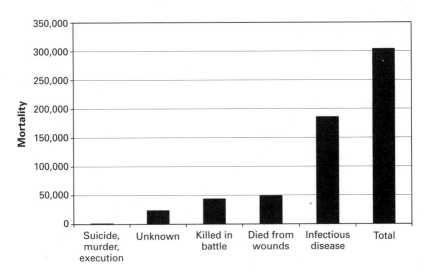

Figure 7.5
Causes of death, American Civil War. Source: J. Barnes, *The Medical and Surgical History of the War of the Rebellion (1861–5)*, vols. 1–3 (US Army, 1870–1888).

and so (aside from anecdotal records) we have little empirical evidence to indicate which specific pathogens accounted for what proportion of that aggregate mortality.

Such problems of co-infection persist into the modern era. According to Grant and Jorgenson, who studied the mortality patterns of Soviet troops in Afghanistan during the 1980s, disease played a significant role in mortality. Specifically, they report that less than 3 percent of casualties resulted directly from combat, yet approximately 76 percent of Soviet casualties resulted from infectious diseases, including malaria, plague, typhus, hepatitis, and various forms of dysentery.[86]

Civil War and Disease as Public Bads

The economist Paul Collier notes that collapsed states, often as the result of civil war, act as the epicenters of disease and regional turbulence.[87] In this sense, state failure can be also seen as a public bad, which then generates further externalities such as pathogens, which may then function to afflict a specific region, or indeed come to burden the entire world. Toole et al. comment that the civil war in Bosnia during the early 1990s "revealed extensive disruption to basic health services, displacement of more than 1 million Bosnians, severe food shortages in Muslim enclaves in eastern Bosnia, and widespread destruction of public water and sanitation systems. War-related violence remains the most important public health risk; civilians on all sides of the conflict have been intentional targets of physical and sexual violence."[88] Moreover, the extensive empirical analysis of Ghobarah confirms that contiguous civil wars are significantly associated with the spread of HIV in neighboring territories.[89] Furthermore, Garenneand et al. argue that during the civil war in Central Mozambique in the 1990s "mortality from infectious diseases increased dramatically during the civil war."[90] Interestingly, Ghobarah concludes that "the most common impact [of civil war] is through infectious diseases. . . . In fact, by t value, five of the 25 groups most impacted by civil wars are from the increased incidence of malaria. The three other most affected disease groups are tuberculosis, respiratory infections, and other infectious diseases. . . ."[91]

Refugees and Displaced Persons

Civil wars in the modern era are associated with generating significant flows of refugees and internally displaced persons. Since the mid 1980s, the turbulent Western Upper Nile region of the Sudan has seen the emergence of epidemic visceral leishmaniasis, and massive mortality of the local population. Seaman et al. note that the epidemic began in 1983, when the civil war between the Nilotic peoples of the South and the Arab-African populations of the North began again in earnest, as a result of the introduction of the parasite through troop vectors from its regions of endemicity. This low-intensity but protracted civil war has resulted in complete disruption of the health-care infrastructure in the area, in increased malnutrition, and in huge population movements of both combatants and civilians. According to Seaman, "movement to escape the fighting and to search for food . . . has probably increased the rate of transmission and facilitated the spread of the epidemic within [the western upper Nile region] and beyond. Agriculture and cattle rearing have been disrupted by the war, resulting in more persistent malnutrition which has probably contributed to a higher conversion rate to clinical disease . . . and hence to high mortality."[92] Moreover, the hostilities have disrupted both coherent epidemiological surveillance of the epidemic and the provision of treatment to the infected, as expatriate medical staff are often evacuated because of the fighting.[93] As a result, this conflict-induced epidemic has resulted in catastrophic mortality throughout the region: "Between 38 percent and 58 percent of the population reportedly died, and up to 70 percent in the most affected areas. . . . 80,000–136,000 people who might otherwise have been expected to live, have died since 1984."[94]

Rey et al. note that refugees returning to Kosovo after the conflict with the Serbs in 1998 generated an epidemic of hepatitis (HAV and HEV, specifically) in that region.[95] The displacement of populations as a result of civil war has also been associated with recent outbreaks of epidemic typhus in sub-Saharan Africa. According to the epidemiologists J. Ndihokubwayo and D. Raoult, Burundi's lengthy civil war of 1993–2006 forced a significant proportion of the population to "live in the cold, promiscuity, and malnutrition of makeshift refugee camps." They conclude that "political unrest as well as numerous civil wars are now epidemiological factors favor[ing] outbreaks of epidemic typhus at any time."[96] Toole and Waldman concur, noting that war generates conditions of stress, malnourishment, lack of sanitary facilities, and lack of access to public health provision that contribute directly to the spread of communicable diseases within densely populated refugee camps.[97] Ghobarah concurs:

Prolonged and bloody civil wars are likely to displace large populations, either internally or as refugees. Epidemic diseases—tuberculosis, measles, pneumonia, cholera, typhoid, paratyphoid, and dysentery—are likely to emerge from crowding, bad water, and poor sanitation in camps, while malnutrition and stress compromise people's immune systems. [Furthermore] the camps become vectors for transmitting disease to other regions. Prevention and treatment programs already weakened by the destruction of health-care infrastructure during civil wars become overwhelmed as new strains of infectious disease bloom. For example, efforts to eradicate Guinea worm, river blindness, and polio—successful in most countries—have been severely disrupted in states experiencing the most severe civil wars.[98]

Smallman-Raynor and Cliff conclude that civil war can affect the spread of epidemic disease through various mechanisms of diffusion: "... the population movements engendered by the Cuban Insurrection (1895–98) and the Philippine-American War (1899–1902) were found to be associated with a strengthening of the geographical corridors of epidemic transmission that would ordinarily be witnessed in peacetime."[99] Przeworski et al. argue that political disruption generates persistent and negative effects on economic growth rates in affected polities.[100] Thus, the economic shortfall induced by political instability typically results in a reduction of government revenues available for expenditure on public goods such as health care, clean water, and sanitation, which in turn greatly facilitates the proliferation of pathogens in a society. The pernicious effects of war on capital (both fiscal and human), particularly as they affect the provision of public health, are very much in need of further empirical investigation.

War may be seen as malign not only in and of itself but also in its role as the progenitor and disseminator of disease. Consequently, war should be understood as amplifying disease through its contribution to contagion as a function of emergent properties. Thus, even regional wars may generate the circumstances for pathogenic emergence (and further evolution) that contribute to the spread of global public bads in the form of pandemic diseases. "If we fail to recognize the evolutionary changes in pathogen virulence that our activities may inadvertently cause," Ewald warns, "then we will pay the price in sickness and death not just until our activities change the environment back to a state that favors the benign forms, but rather until the evolutionary change toward benignness is completed."[101] Collectively, such preliminary evidence reinforces the hypothesis that war and disease may operate synergistically as symbiotic externalities wherein the former extensively reinforces the latter, with this malign nexus operating at domestic, regional, and global levels.

In summation, the following factors, generated or exacerbated by conflict, contribute directly to the emergence and/or proliferation of pathogens:

- increased population density (combatants and civilian)
- famine-induced malnourishment, compromising immunity
- conflict-related mobility or vectors (troops and refugees)
- lack of hygienic conditions (water, etc.)
- destruction of health infrastructure
- lack of access to health services
- impediments to treatment
- poverty (induced or exacerbated)
- inhibition of effective public health surveillance
- sexual coercion and commercial sex
- physical and psychological stress, compromising host immunity.

8

On Health, Power, and Security

History of the Debate on Health Security

The role of infectious disease in modern security studies originates in the historical accounts of Thucydides, Machiavelli, and Rousseau, all regarded as republican progenitors of the political paradigm known as Classical Realism. Deudney has argued that Realism as a theoretical construct (along with its cousin Liberalism) is derivative of an earlier "republican" tradition, with both terms coined in the nineteenth century.[1] Historians have continued this discourse on contagion into the modern era, noting the profound influence of pathogens on the course of history, and in certain cases the fate of countries.[2]

As was argued above, the republican political tradition (with its Realist and Liberal descendents) constitutes the theoretical antecedent for those political scientists who began their inquiries in the mid 1990s, including Dennis Pirages and the present author.[3] Pirages was the first to assert that infectious disease constituted a direct threat to human security insofar as it places the security of individuals and communities over that of states:

Infectious diseases are potentially the largest threat to human security lurking in the post-Cold War world. Emerging from the Cold War era, it is understandably difficult to reprogram security thinking to take account of non-military threats. But a new focus that included microsecurity issues could lead to interesting cost-benefit thinking. In the short term, policymakers need to understand the potential seriousness of the problem and reallocate resources accordingly.[4]

The nascent field of "health security" enjoyed a pronounced increase in salience during 2000, when the US National Intelligence Council issued a National Intelligence Estimate which concluded that infectious disease posed both direct and indirect threats to the material interests and security of the United States (Gordon 2000). In that report, the NIC stated:

New and reemerging infectious diseases will . . . complicate US and global security over the next 20 years. These diseases will endanger US citizens at home and abroad, threaten armed forces deployed overseas, and exacerbate social and political instability in key countries and regions in which the United States has significant interests.[5]

Subsequently, based on the recommendations of the National Security Council, the Clinton administration declared HIV/AIDS a threat to global security.[6] On January 10, 2000, Vice-President Al Gore articulated the Clinton administration's position that HIV/AIDS constituted a significant threat to global security in an address to the UN Security Council:

For the nations of sub-Saharan Africa, AIDS is not just a humanitarian crisis. It is a security crisis—because it threatens not just individual citizens, but the very institutions that define and defend the character of a society. This disease weakens workforces and saps economic strength. It strikes at the military, and subverts the forces of order and peacekeeping. AIDS is one of the most devastating threats ever to confront the world community. Many have called the battle against it a sacred crusade. The United Nations was created to stop wars. Now, we must wage and win a great and peaceful war of our time—the war against AIDS.[7]

Such perceptions of the gravity of the AIDS crisis persisted into the early months of the George W. Bush administration, and were echoed by Secretary of State Colin Powell on June 25, 2001 in an address to the UN General Assembly. Powell also framed the issue as one of national security: "I was a soldier and I know of no enemy in war more insidious or vicious than AIDS, an enemy that poses a clear and present danger to the world. . . ."[8] Under-Secretary of State Paula Dobriansky concurred: "HIV/AIDS is a threat to security and global stability, plain and simple."[9]

On July 17, 2000, under the leadership of US Ambassador Richard Holbrooke, the UN Security Council adopted Resolution 1308 (2000), which explicitly declared the HIV/AIDS pandemic a threat to global security. This was the first time (in the modern era) that an issue of public health had been elevated to such status, and it illustrated the continuing transformation in thinking about new threats to security in the new millennium. This recognition of the centrality of health to issues of power and security was profoundly disturbing to the Galenists who had worked for decades to create the false dichotomization of health and security.

Regrettably, this dramatic resurrection of the salience of global public health issues, and their influence on security debates, was subsequently derailed by several factors. First, the attacks of September 11 fundamentally transformed the intellectual space of the post-Cold War security rubric, as terrorism was thereafter defined as the principal and immediate direct threat to the security of the United States. Unfortunately, the human tendency to fix on one proximate threat while ignoring others, so dominant during the Cold War, rose to the fore again in the post-9/11 era. Other process-based threats, including environmental destruction, resource scarcity, and contagion, were shunted aside. The novel terror-induced myopia that gripped Washington was further augmented by the anthrax attacks. These biological attacks in particular succeeded in framing the health-security debate primarily through the lens of bioterrorism, and US funding became increasingly directed toward biodefense initiatives (e.g., Biowatch and Bioshield) and away from investments in basic public health infrastructure. In addition, long-simmering tensions between Secretary of State Powell and Secretary of Defense Rumsfeld resulted in the gradual marginalization of the Department of State, of its key players, and of its more nuanced and holistic conceptualizations of global security, which included threats to public health.

In 2002, several political scientists (Elbe, Ostergard, Peterson, Price-Smith, Singer) analyzed the validity of the hypothesis that infectious disease represented a security concern. Within this larger debate, the threat posed by HIV/AIDS has received the greatest amount of attention, producing much heat and some light. Stefan Elbe argued, convincingly, that the deliberate transmission of HIV, through the horrid practice of war-rape, was widely employed by military forces throughout sub-Saharan Africa.[10] Robert Ostergard exposed the palpable Western ethnocentrism of security studies, and argued that infectious disease constituted a significant direct threat to the security of numerous polities throughout the developing world.[11] Peter Singer argued that "the looming security implications of AIDS, particularly within Africa, are now a baseline assumption. AIDS not only threatens to heighten the risks of war, but also multiplies its impact."[12] Susan Peterson examined the claims of health security theorists and concluded that they possessed a certain degree of validity, although she argued (correctly) that disease had a greater potential for the internal destabilization of states than for fomenting wars between sovereign states.[13]

In 2003, the RAND analysts Jennifer Brower and Peter Chalk also noted the insidious nature of the disease threat to US national security. They argued that "disease acts as a highly pervasive influence that not only impinges on security in terms of traditional conceptions of state stability, but, more insidiously, directly undermines and weakens the essential socioeconomic foundations upon which an effective polity ultimately depends."[14] Therefore contagion might operate to destabilize those poorer countries that exhibit low levels of capacity, and the resulting negative externalities might then radiate on a regional and global scale, undermining the interests of the great powers.

The SARS epidemic of 2002–03 certainly had the biological potential to evolve into a security threat, and that potential was perceived by China's political elites (Huang 2003). After the SARS scare, linkages between HIV/AIDS, domestic level governance, and security were explored,[15] and sporadic attempts to link infectious disease and security have followed in recent years.[16] Unfortunately, advocates of the health and security debate have recently encountered resistance from the Galenic community and from orthodox security theorists who remain wedded to the "guns, bombs, and terror" paradigm and reject unconventional process-based threats such as environmental destruction.[17]

On Health and Power

The historical literature clearly indicates that the policy elites of earlier generations understood the connectivity between the health of the population and the prosperity, cohesion, and power of the state. The concept of political power was effectively articulated by Hans Morgenthau: "When we speak of power we mean man's control over the minds and actions of other men. By political power we refer to the mutual relations of control among the holders of public authority and between the latter and the people at large. Political power is (therefore) a psychological relation between those who exercise it and those over whom it is exercised."[18]

If disease is the antithesis of health, then periodic manifestations of contagion should, logically, impoverish and destabilize the state and diminish its power relative to unaffected polities. Variance in the magnitude of such disruption is dependent on several things, including the lethality and transmissibility of the specific pathogen, the capacity and resilience of the state, and the human ecology of the affected society (including levels of acquired immunity). Thus, it is not surprising that population health was understood as a central component of state power, and particularly hard power, which explains the development of contagionist practices to counter the ineffective practices of the Galenic school. Thus, the policy community has correctly regarded infectious disease as corrosive of socio-political cohesion, economic prosperity, and puissance.

The concept of power (in the domain of health and security) possesses two faces, with the first face being the power of the state with respect to the population over which it presides. As was argued above, contagion may produce disintegration of social capital and cohesion, a rise in identity-based violence between factions (based on ethnicity or class), and an erosion of domestic productivity and prosperity, that collectively threatens the material interests of political elites and the integrity of state institutions. Consonant with the dictates of contagionist doctrine the state (in order to preserve order, its material interests, and its survival) may consequently engage in coercive practices against its own people. Such abuses of power by the state against society are well documented herein, ranging from the draconian practices of the Mantuan and Florentine lords to the *Medizinalpolizei* of Imperial Prussia, and in modern times, the Mugabe regime in Zimbabwe.

The second face of power emanates from the material reality that manifestations of epidemic disease clearly have the ability to weaken a state relative to its sovereign rivals. Epidemics may visit destruction on a state's apparatus of coercion (military and police forces), kill important personnel in the bureaucracy, constrain and erode economic prosperity and thereby diminish the base of tax revenues, and undermine the cohesion of the state. Collectively, these effects will vary according to the particular attributes of the pathogen, immunity of population, state capacity, co-infection, and even geography.[19] For example, a state that is simultaneously burdened by a number of various pathogens (say, malaria, HIV, and schistosomiasis) that afflict a significant proportion of the population (>20 percent per annum) will be much weaker than a state in which similarly malign pathogens are less prevalent and the burden of disease is therefore much lower.[20] Thus, over the decades, the power of the second state relative to the first will increase substantially.

Thucydides clearly understood this negative association between disease and power. The arrival of "the plague" clearly undermined the socio-political cohesion of the Athenian polity, generated lawlessness and disorder, and destroyed circa 30 percent of the empire's infantry. The contagion resulted in the death of leading members of the state, most notably Pericles, after which the rise of demagogues led eventually to the defeat of Athens. Machiavelli's account of the Black Death as it visited Firenze (Florence) also illustrates the destructive effects of the plague on effective governance and social cohesion.[21]

Thus, modern conceptualizations of health and security emanate from the republican political tradition, and its descendent Realism, which emphasizes state survival through the maximization of power. Realist theory stipulates that the state will act in its own material self-interests, or in the interests of those dominant factions that constitute and/or control the machinery of the state. The theory also assumes that the international system is anarchical, and that the condition of competitive anarchy precludes significant cooperation between states unless such cooperation is in their own material and/or ideational self-interest. This hegemonic theory explains the evolution of international public health regimes (such as the International Health Regulations) as purely derivative of the material interests of the great powers.[22] Hegemonic theories of regime formation and evolution also help to explain the rapid revision of the International Health Regulations in the wake of SARS. Given that health was historically recognized as a fulcrum of state power, and subsequently as a tool of imperial expansion, international health regimes followed in order to perpetuate the dominance of the powers that had crafted them. The medical historian George Rosen argues that during the era of mercantilism, wherein the consolidation of the modern state took place, "the welfare of society was regarded as identical with the welfare of the state." He continues:

Since power was considered the first interest of the state, most elements of mercantilist policy were advanced and justified as strengthening the power of the realm. *Raison d'etat* was the fulcrum of social policy. As the rulers and their advisers saw it, what was required was first of all a large population; second, that the population be provided for in a material sense; and thirdly, that it should be under the control of government so that it could be turned to whatever use public policy required. (I)t was recognized everywhere in some degree that effective use of population within a country required attention to problems of health.[23]

In the early to mid 1600s, the collection of data and the use of science (including medicine) to bolster the power of the state was the domain of "political arithmeticians" such as William Petty and John Graunt. They used the emerging science of statistics to quantify the burdens of illness to the economy and state power.[24] In the 1620s, Prussia's political elite explicitly recognized the centrality of population health to state power and established the *Medizinalpolizei* (medical police). From 1655 on, the association between health and power was promulgated throughout Prussia by the political administrator Veit Ludwig von Seckendorff. According to von Seckendorff, the state was obliged to establish laws to ensure the well-being of the population, such that their number and the productivity of the citizenry would increase, generating prosperity and thus puissance for the nation.[25] The historian John Hays concurs:

Early modern European states gradually came to recognize connections between the size of their populations and both military power and economic prosperity. . . . Enlightened despots of the same period embarked on programs of "medical police," particularly attending to the control of epidemics through isolation and quarantines. . . . The concern that eighteenth-century states manifested for the health of their soldiers and sailors suggests the importance of the military motive for such benevolent behavior.[26]

It was during this period that medicine and public health, with their increasing capacity to control disease, became effective tools of imperial expansion for the European powers. Medical and sanitary advances augmented the ability of European forces to withstand hostile foreign disease environments. Such technological advances also conferred symbolic and psychological advantages on European forces: they were perceived as masters over illness. The demographer Philip Curtin posits that European forces benefited enormously from this "revolution in tropical medicine and hygiene," which permitted and augmented an unprecedented projection of European power into tropical regions.[27] This association between health and hard power intensified in the aftermath of the Franco-Prussian War as universal conscription became ubiquitous throughout the European states. Thus, a direct and positive association emerged between the sheer size of the population, their health and productivity, and the projection of martial power.[28]

Moreover, the domestic institutional architecture created by states to contain epidemic disease during the early years of the Westphalian era (1648–present) suggests a desire to preserve both societal order and state power through legal mechanisms of disease containment. Such mechanisms included the Bavarian law that made smallpox vaccination compulsory in 1807—a law that was emulated by Denmark (1810), Russia (1812), and Sweden (1816).[29] Britain enacted similar health regulations to preserve state power and prosperity—notably the Contagious Diseases Acts of 1864,[30] which "licensed and controlled prostitution in an attempt to preserve the health of the military."[31]

(Re-)Defining Security

Given the centrality of health to the cohesion, wealth, and power of the state, widely accepted by political elites in prior generations, why should health have been de-securitized in the modern era (1945–present)? Opponents of the "health and security" paradigm approach the issue as if the association had simply appeared *ex nihilo*, ignoring the wealth of historical sources that document the lineage of the relationship.[32] However, the securitization of health is not novel at all, but hearkens back to a classical (republican) vein of thought that pervades the discipline of political science and its various subdisciplines.[33]

In 1983, the political scientist Richard Ullman redefined security in a manner that transcended those modern Realist definitions that focus exclusively on military threats, arguing that "defining national security in purely military terms conveys a profoundly false image of reality [and] causes states to concentrate on military threats and to ignore other and more harmful dangers."[34] Further, Ullman defined a threat to national security as "an action or sequence of events that (1) threatens drastically and over a relatively brief span of time to degrade the quality of life for the inhabitants of a state, or (2) threatens significantly to narrow the range of policy choices available to the government of a state or to private, non-governmental entities (persons, groups, corporations) within the state."[35] This redefinition of security is useful in that it includes material-contextual factors, and thus non-military threats—e.g., the destruction of a state's population by a pathogenic agent such as avian influenza, or the human immunodeficiency virus (HIV). Furthermore, Ullman's definition places emphasis on processes as threats, not just on human enemies. This represents an important intellectual advance because processes can compromise security over very long periods of time, and are therefore rather difficult to observe. As a species, humans suffer from a truncated attention span, and an event (e.g., a bombing in the London subway) is sure to capture the attention of the global media, and thus policy elites. Attenuated processes (e.g., global climate shifts or HIV-induced destruction of populations) are much more difficult to observe. Such malignant processes suffer from reduced saliency until some critical threshold (or tipping point) is reached, whereupon macro-level non-linear destabilization occurs and the media and policy makers are forced to deal with the issue. The emergence of the hole in the ozone layer over the Antarctic region illustrates this problem. In this particular case, satellite-procured data on strato-spheric ozone concentrations was delivered to an array of sophisticated computers for analysis. The computers were programmed to detect linear changes in the concentration of ozone, such that when rapid and non-linear decay in the ozone layer was observed, it was dismissed by the computer programs as an error in the data and disregarded for several years.[36]

A second challenge to orthodox militaristic conceptualizations of secu-rity came from Barry Buzan, who argued that national security encom-passes various spheres of activity including military, economic, political, societal, and environmental dimensions.[37] Furthermore, he understood the complex and interactive effects that each domain could exert on the others, and therefore his conceptions are holistic. Buzan argued that "individual national securities can only be fully understood when con-sidered in relations both to each other and to larger patterns of relations in the system as a whole."[38]

Additional challenges to the militaristic paradigm came from Edward Kolodziej[39] and from Kalevi Holsti. Holsti expressed dismay at the disci-pline's pronounced dislocation from the empirical reality faced by the majority of countries, echoing claims of disciplinary ethnocentrism.[40] According to Holsti, "strategic studies continue to be seriously divorced from the practices of war. . . . The argument . . . is that security *between* states in the Third World . . . and elsewhere has become increasingly dependent on security *within* those states. The trend is clear: the threat of war between countries is receding, while the incidence of vio-lence within states is on an upward curve."[41] Therefore, endogenous threats[42] to prosperity, cohesion, and power may in fact present greater threats to many countries than the martial power of their contiguous neighbors.

The emergence of the environmental-security debate in the early 1990s provided for additional definitions of security that departed from the orthodox military-centric viewpoint.[43] Indeed, early conceptualizations of the health security paradigm noted the profound connectivity between environmental change and pathogenic emergence, proliferation, and mutation (Price-Smith 2002). The destruction that Hurricane Katrina visited on New Orleans (and proximate areas) in 2005 exposed the vulnerability of the sovereign state, and the people it is obliged to protect, to non-military threats. Despite the policy-making community's increasing recognition of naturally occurring threats to the state, the academic community has been exceptionally slow to recognize the threat posed by such material-contextual phenomena, which include infectious agents.

Issues of public health, then, exhibit a significant impact on the state precisely because of their historical relations to power and order, and because diseases have the potential to kill a great proportion of the population, deplete state coffers, destabilize the polity, and weaken the state relative to its rivals. An infectious disease may constitute a direct and/or an indirect threat to a state's coherence, prosperity, and power. Thus, it is entirely logical to extol the virtues of investing in population health and, simultaneously, to maintain a republican state-centric view of security. The state is thus motivated by enlightened self-interest to protect its power base, which by extension entails protecting the health of its people from pathogens.

The modern health-security debate remains impoverished on several counts. First, the arguments against securitization presented by Roger Cooter and others are often profoundly ahistorical and largely ideological. Moreover, the current debate over the securitization of infectious disease (most of which focuses on the HIV pandemic) appears to begin in the late 1980s, after the diagnosis of AIDS. The imposition of such severe temporal restrictions on the debate results in a discourse that largely ignores the connectivity between infectious disease, governments and their constitutive institutions, and civil society over thousands of years of recorded history. The ignorance of basic principles of public health, epidemiology, and microbiology by certain social scientists participating in the debate is also deleterious to the construction of any serious debate of the issues. Similarly, the ignorance of political and economic thought by many in the medical community limits thoughtful debate on the issue. In addition, the securitization of disease should in no way be focused exclusively on the effects of one pathogen, even one as pernicious as HIV. There are many pathogens that possess the capacity to inflict great physical harm on a population (particularly influenza), and which also threaten economic productivity and global trade (e.g., SARS). To limit the debate to HIV/AIDS excludes an entire spectrum of other possible threats to prosperity, stability, and power, and it is analytically problematic.

Furthermore, the designation of a pathogen as a threat to "health security" will vary to some degree from one sovereign entity to another, as different polities will exhibit different vulnerabilities, based on the population's genetic or acquired resistance levels, state capacity, geographic location, etc. Thus, the Western bias of the security literature is problematic, such that a phenomenon is typically not seen as a threat to national security unless it constitutes a threat to the security of the hegemon (in this case, the United States). The abstract concept of health security should surely apply to all sovereign states. Thus, it is nonsense to say that a pathogen does not qualify as a threat to the security of a country simply because it is not a direct threat to the United States, and such discourse reflects both Western hubris and muddled thinking. If an epidemic were to break out in a country that possessed low capacity, and therefore low resilience, and overwhelm the population, it might indeed constitute a direct threat to that country's security. However, that same pathogen might not represent a threat to a member of the G-8, whose members possess significant endogenous capacity, and a different configuration of the human ecology. Thus, it seems reasonable to postulate that a pathogen such as HIV constitutes a qualitatively greater threat to the least-developed countries that possess less resilience.

Conversely, certain pathogens possess various genetic attributes and adaptations that allow them to thrive in the environments of the developed world but not in impoverished environments. For example, SARS presented a clear threat to China and Hong Kong (and Canada) because it thrived within the air conditioning and sanitation systems of modern buildings, whereas it was easily contained in the low-tech but open-air hospitals of Viet Nam.[44] Therefore, prosperity (in the form of high-tech buildings equipped with air conditioning can, in perverse fashion, enable different pathogens that thrive in those particular ecological niches. Ultimately, the security calculus must be pathogen-specific, moderated by a country's capacity and ecological configuration.

Moreover, as Marshall McLuhan predicted, advances in technology, such as the increasing speed of travel and telecommunications, have created a "global village."[45] These accelerating processes of "globalization" have greatly increased the scale of connectivity between the developed and the developing countries, such that destabilization in one country can trigger a non-linear global chain reaction of disruption. The Asian financial crisis of 1997 is an excellent illustration of such global connectivity, as the economic destabilization of Thailand ultimately led to profound turbulence in the markets and economies of distal countries, including Russia and Brazil. In the domain of infectious disease, this means that the emergence of a new lethal pathogen in South Asia (e.g., SARS), can trigger fear and anxiety, leading to the rapid destabilization of markets throughout the Pacific Rim.

Further, as September 11 illustrated quite vividly, instability in the developing countries can directly affect the security interests of the developed countries. If disease stresses the capacity of a polity, it may interact with other variables in complex and non-linear fashion to contribute to the erosion of effective governance, resulting in weak or collapsed states. Furthermore, if a pathogen destabilizes the economy and political cohesion of a certain country, the collapsed state may subsequently generate externalities that indirectly undermine the interests (and the security) of the great powers. Weak and collapsed states are breeding grounds for the disaffected and may become harbors for radical groups (such as Al-Qaeda) seeking to inflict destruction on the dominant sovereign states. In this fashion, disease-induced instability in developing countries may indirectly threaten the national security of many developed states (including the United States).

There is evidence that disease may certainly facilitate internal turbulence, but is there solid evidence that imbalances in power generated by contagion will produce war between sovereign states? To date, the balance of evidence suggests that there appears to be no positive association between the incidence of disease and subsequent war between sovereign states.[46] Despite the Realist axiom that asymmetries or shifts in relative power between sovereign states contribute to conflict between those powers, this association does not appear to hold when one state is severely afflicted by disease. One explanation for this is that pathogens may afflict geographically contiguous states to an equivalent extent, and contagion appears to have a sclerotic or paralytic effect on both societies and the institutions of the state (including the apparatus of coercion). Therefore, in the face of contagion, the state's institutional capacity to act in a bellicose manner is consequently reduced, even though the relative power of country B may begin to exceed that of country A as a result of the contagion. Second, if country A is besieged with contagion and country B is less afflicted, it makes little rational sense for country B to invade country A and thereby expose its soldiers to the epidemic, taking the additional risk that said troops could then bring the pathogen back to country B on their demobilization. Thus, epidemic disease may significantly inhibit the operational capacity of military units, generate the rational calculus that conflict should be avoided, and thereby force a cessation of hostilities or inhibit the initiation of conflict. In that manner the war/disease relationship may operate on occasion as a negative feedback loop wherein military conflict initially acts as a disease amplifier, and thereafter the spread of infection within military units intensifies until they lose the capacity to prosecute their campaigns.

Republican Realism

. . . the central theme of international relations is not evil but tragedy.
—Robert Jervis[47]

Given that modern strains of Realism are the descendents of republican political thought, I argue for a republican revision of Realism. Realism's historical focus on survival, (which emanates from republican theory) as the ultimate goal of the state remains in effect, as all states seek to perpetuate their existence to some degree. The quest for survival therefore entails the maximization of power, in order to dissuade other competitors from undertaking hostile action against the state. This maximization of power entails the protection of the people, from whom the state derives its prosperity and its military power. Indeed, prosperity is central to military power, as economic assets are fungible and may be readily translated into purchases of advanced weapons systems, training of skilled personnel, and materiel. The protection of the people from pathogens is also central to the maintenance of order within the polity, ensuring that state institutions continue to function with a moderate degree of efficacy and that the state and the society do not fragment internally.

However, the utility of certain tenets of modern Realism must now be questioned. First, as the political scientists Graham Allison and Randall Schweller concede, the state is not a unitary, monolithic actor,[48] as various factions (i.e., interest groups) or organizations within the state (i.e., bureaucratic divisions) compete for fiscal resources and to project their particular interests during the processes of foreign policy formation.[49] The second major shortcoming of the Rational Actor Model is that it assumes that a state acts (as one entity) to make the most rational decisions possible, therefore maximizing its power and its interests. Such assumptions of rationality are certainly questionable in the domain of health and foreign policy, and the political scientist Stephen Walt has extensively criticized assumptions of rationality in game-theoretical decision making.[50]

As seen throughout the case studies, the assumption of rational maximization of utility by the state, in dealing with other international actors and/or dealing with its own population, is questionable. In the cases of BSE, SARS, and HIV/AIDS, sovereign states have engaged in trade embargoes driven by fear and uncertainty, have restricted the movements of both trade goods and human personnel, have sought to obscure the magnitude of contagion from the international community, have denied the problem, and have resisted cooperating with other international actors until compelled to do so. The case of the 1918 pandemic influenza is difficult to characterize, as the war precluded cooperation between many of the infected parties and the protagonists applied draconian restrictions on reporting the contagion. However, even among non-combatants there was little cooperation on the issue, although this probably was due to the fact that medicine and public health were incapable of providing effective prophylaxis, let alone treatment.

As I argued above, psychological elements, such as perception (or misperception), emotion, concepts of group identity, and image theory, have figured in the evolution of epidemics and in the magnification of their associated externalities. Such a republican revision of Realism echoes the work of Robert Jervis, who, as a proponent of Realism, nonetheless realized the importance of psychological effects on the (mis)perceptions and calculations of policy elites. It is imperative to recognize that the empirical biological reality of epidemics is moderated by perceptions, by affect (emotion), by concepts of identity, and by bounded rationality. Only when we begin to engage in a republican synthesis of the paradigms of Realism and political psychology do we gain any significant analytical traction in the realm of health and security studies. The trans-national character of the threat complicates our ability to perceive it accurately, and the uncertainty associated with novel pathogens complicates our assessment of the risk. This makes it exceedingly difficult for political elites to gauge the level of the threat accurately.

The globalization of pathogens generates additional complexities for orthodox conceptualizations of Realism, which stipulates that states will engage in strategies of self-help to contain pathogens within their borders. Such containment may require sealing borders to trade and migration, mass quarantining of infected individuals, and continued effective surveillance. Obviously, many states (including the US) lack the endogenous capacity for surveillance, diagnosis, effective prophylaxis and treatment, and means of quarantine and border control. That said, states may thus find it expedient to engage in compacts to provide mutual assistance as based on their perceived self-interest. In this sense, the emergence and evolution of global health regimes merely reflects the historical interests of the hegemonic power (or a coalition of great powers) in containing those specific pathogens that threatened the interests of those states. Thus, the threat of contagion establishes the republican basis for inter-state cooperation as a means to protect the material interests of all states.

Republican theory permits the reform of Realism to explain the behavior of states in the domain of infectious disease. First, we must abandon assumptions of the state as a unitary actor. As witnessed in the case of China during the SARS scare, different segments of the bureaucracy impede the effective flow of information to the apex of government. Further, competition between domestic institutions certainly undermined rational responses by federal governments in the case of BSE, ranging from the persistent incompetence of the Ministry of Agriculture, Fisheries and Food in Britain to the influence of domestic agricultural lobbies on the efficacy of the Department of Agriculture in the United States. Moreover, despite the rhetoric of free trade in the modern era, the BSE crisis has served as an excuse for protectionist behavior.

Furthermore, decision makers exhibit bounded rationality, which stipulates that they will attempt to make the most rational decision possible but face considerable constraints.[51] Such constraints include serious difficulties in the estimation of risk, particularly in the face of a novel and emergent pathogen of unknown etiology and lethality. Time constraints will also limit the generation of accurate information regarding the etiology, lethality, and transmissibility of said pathogen, further impeding optimal decision making. Such limited information results in significant uncertainty, which in turn can generate significant manifestations of anxiety, even fear, and which often leads to overreaction. As Jervis argued, the incapacity to perceive threats accurately often leads to

Pareto-suboptimal decision making.[52] Conversely, decision makers may also seek cognitive consistency (by reinterpreting or disregarding information that conflicts with their existing belief structures), and may engage in excessive minimization or denial of a threat.[53] Furthermore, humans exhibit the tendency to perceive threats as "enemies" and not as "processes." Security theorists should be aware of such cognitive biases and should understand that threats to both national and international security can take the form of long-term, complex, and non-linear processes.

A republican reformation of Realism maintains that sovereign states remain the dominant actors in the system, and that international regimes (e.g., the IHR) merely reflect the power and interests of a dominant state or coalition of states. However, republican Realism notes that threats to security can emanate from non-military sources, such as non-state actors (terrorists), or from processes such as pathogenic emergence. Moreover, the Realist dichotomization of the domestic and systems levels of analysis is problematic, given that the breakdown of governance within a sovereign state can generate radiating externalities that compromise the security of proximate states. The discipline of security studies must abandon its ethnocentrism and recognize that the immiseration of peoples in the developing world, and the collapse of governance therein, presents a novel threat to the security of the developed nations as well. Thus, republican theory, with its emphasis on *physis*, embraces the concept of complex interdependence in the human ecology, and notes that the natural world maintains a profound capacity to influence the conduct of human affairs.

Mechanisms

In sum, infectious disease operates in a number of ways to destabilize a state from within or to weaken a state to the extent that its ability to project power, and indeed to defend itself, is significantly compromised. The balance of evidence suggests that contagion does not start wars between sovereign states (although it does seem to possess the historical capacity to immobilize military forces, and could thereby result in a cessation of hostilities).

At the domestic level, infectious disease acts to undermine state capacity, and therefore the stability of the polity, through the following mechanisms:

Mortality and morbidity Disease-induced death and debilitation deplete the endogenous base of human capital, undercut the productivity of workers, and generate negative effects at the micro, sectoral, and macro levels of the economy. The destruction of the population also compromises military recruitment, and generates the loss of skilled personnel.

Declining ingenuity Disease-induced erosion of human capital limits a society's capacity to generate ingenuity, eroding downstream social and technical innovation, impeding economic productivity, and undercutting the state's resilience (ability to respond to crises).

Diminished revenue Disease-induced declines in productivity result in economic contraction that will consequently limit the tax revenues and other resources that are extracted from the people by the state. As the tax base erodes, the capacity of the state to provide public goods for its own citizens declines correspondingly, as does its ability to project martial power.

Reduced social capital Disease generates in/out group behavior, results in the stigmatization of infecteds and/or vectors, and generates hostility between ethnic groups and/or classes. This generates destabilization within the polity and thereby undercuts the stability of the state as a macro entity.

Reduced legitimacy Widespread contagion may induce economic contraction, and cause the provision of public services to decline.[54] State institutions may become increasingly brittle and sclerotic. The people may then see the state as ineffective and in violation of the social contract. Collectively, this may foster perceptions of the state as increasingly illegitimate, and thereby exacerbate internal social destabilization. Ultimately, the state may retaliate in draconian fashion against its own people (as in modern Zimbabwe).

Changes in relative power The destruction of important personnel throughout the bureaucracy, and the apparatus of coercion (i.e., the military and police forces), will jeopardize the state's ability to protect itself from external aggression. Further, the erosion of the state's fiscal resources will limit its ability to project power abroad and its ability to defend itself in the face of aggression. Such changes in relative power may affect downstream relations between states after the contagion has passed.

Connectivity As a result of the increasing interdependence resulting from accelerating globalization, the interests of the great powers are now profoundly linked to processes and events occurring in developing countries, such that destabilization of a polity in Central Asia can lead to externalities that directly affect and undermine the security of the United Kingdom. Thus, disease-induced destabilization in one region may compromise the prosperity and the security of all.

Furthermore, I argue, certain pathogens constitute significant and perhaps imminent threats to security, whereas other agents do not. For example, the re-emergence of a devastating H1N1 influenza virus, which in 1918 killed 50 million people, crippled armies, destabilized economies, and contributed to sclerotic governance, surely constitutes a direct threat to all countries. Globalization may, in fact, result in a pandemic of even greater scope and perhaps even greater lethality. On the other end of the spectrum is Lyme disease, which is endemic, is not transmissible from human to human, and often can be treated by antibiotic prophylaxis. I find it inconceivable to argue that Lyme disease constitutes a threat to the security of any polity. The following criteria constitute benchmarks for evaluating whether a pathogen constitutes a "security" threat to a given sovereign state:

• The negative health effects produced by the pathogen induce a minimum 1 percent/annum drag on the national GDP.
• The pathogen accounts for the mortality of 1 percent of the total adult population (15–55 years of age) per annum.
• The pathogen results in the severe debilitation of 10 percent of the total adult population per annum.

Doubtless, these criteria will provoke enormous debate among the "health and security" community, and that is my intent.[55]

Conclusion

The complex linkages between public health and conceptualizations of power and security are ancient. They constitute an important historical tradition of republican political thought, having originated during the halcyon days of the Athenian Empire and having enjoyed their heyday from 1348 until the development of antibiotics in the early decades of the twentieth century.[1] Thus, contemporary debates regarding the supposedly recent "securitization" of health issues ignore such historical context.[2] This ignorance of the role of health as a central material-contextual factor obfuscates the relationship between disease, its impacts on society, and the evolution of the sovereign states of Europe. These polities clearly perceived pathogens as profound threats to their material interests, their power, and often their survival.

In view of the profound importance of material-contextual factors in republican thought, I propose a "broadening" of the modern conceptualizations of national security to include non-anthropocentric threats such as environmental destruction, migration, and naturally occurring epidemic disease. Thus, I argue for an analytical focus on "threats" as opposed to "enemies." Such threats may manifest in the form of either temporally constrained events (e.g., the SARS epidemic) or attenuated processes (e.g., the HIV/AIDS pandemic). This distinction is crucial because humans exhibit a psychological tendency to focus on the former, and to ignore the latter, despite the fact that processes may generate powerful long-term negative outcomes for human societies.

Pathogens may constitute a threat to national security through direct and/or indirect impacts on the material interests and the apparatus of the state, which may be moderated to a significant degree by societal and/or contextual factors. The threat presented by contagion is often pathogen-specific, as different pathogenic agents will present variable levels of threat depending on the immunity of the population, the vectors of transmission, and the adaptive capacity of the specific polity involved. Thus, rather than asking whether HIV/AIDS represents a threat to national security, one should ask "Under what specific conditions (viral clade, seroprevalence rate, degree of state capacity, degree of social capital) might HIV/AIDS represent a national security threat to a specific polity (such as Zambia)?" Indeed, I argue specifically that an entire range of infectious diseases, primarily those that kill and debilitate the very young and the very old, are not threats to national security *per se*, although they would certainly constitute issues of human rights and threaten human security. Measles may be a profound issue of human rights, and of economic development, but it does not typically generate mechanisms (demographic, economic, psychological) that undermine the security of the state.[3] Excessively broad categorizations wherein all pathogens are designated as threats to national security must be eschewed because they obfuscate coherent analysis, and because they undermine the credibility of the argument.

What, then, of our original hypotheses about the relations between contagion, the dynamics of state-society interaction, and effects on international governance? The balance of evidence suggests that the following preliminary conclusions may be drawn at this time, as per the domain specified below.

Effects at the Domestic (State) Level

Demographic

Infectious disease may generate significant negative outcomes for human health, ranging from debilitation to the death of the human host. Such outcomes range from a sickened population to widespread mortality and the consequent contraction of the population, or the pathogen-specific contraction of defined age cohorts within a given population. For example, the mortality generated by HIV/AIDS is most pronounced in the 15–45 age cohort. Epidemics may also generate pressures for rapid out-migration from affected areas, as people attempt to flee the source of the infection. Of the case studies, HIV/AIDS exhibits profound negative impacts in the domain of demography, particularly as it continues to destroy entire cohorts of young adults and leaves behind massive orphan populations in a climate of destitution. The global demographic impact of the 1918 pandemic influenza was equally significant (at circa

50 million dead), again with a concentration of mortality in the cohort of young (and previously healthy) adults. Conversely, both the SARS epidemic and the BSE/VCJD epidemics have both exhibited relatively minor levels of morbidity and mortality.

Psychological

The psychological effects of emergent pathogens on the body politic typically include significant levels of uncertainty and difficulties in accurate estimation of risk, contributing to profound emotional responses (notably fear, anxiety, and anger). This affective bias consequently impedes Pareto-optimal rationality. Affective distortions may also facilitate the construction of negative images of the "other," resulting in stigmatization of the ill, persecution of minorities, and diffuse inter-ethnic or inter-class violence. Emotion may also combine with information that conflicts with individual belief structures to generate cognitive dissonance, wherein individuals engage in denial of the discrepant information in order to minimize psychological pain. Of the four modern cases examined herein, both the SARS and BSE epidemics exhibited considerable psychological impacts through the generation of fear, anxiety, and panic and the stigmatization of domestic minorities and foreign populations. The 1918 influenza seems to have had considerable negative effects on the morale of affected military units and on some factions of civil society. The HIV/AIDS pandemic initially provoked considerable fear and anxiety, but in recent years its principal manifestation has taken the form of stigmatization (and often violence) toward the ill. Consequently, any evaluation of pathogenic threats to national security must take into consideration the possible psychological effects of contagion on factions, state-society relations, and material prosperity. Thus, psychological disruptions may trigger disruptions in the realm of the material-contextual.

Economic

Pathogen-induced destruction and/or debilitation of human capital erodes the productivity of workers, imposes direct and indirect costs on families, firms, and the state, and often compromises a society's ability to generate social and technical ingenuity. Given that the burden of disease typically falls on the poorer segments of the population, the proliferation of pathogens may exacerbate or intensify inter-class hostilities as the gap between rich and poor expands under conditions of contagion. Destruction of the endogenous human capital base will therefore compromise micro- and macro-level economic productivity, and may severely impair those sectors of the economy that are labor-intensive (e.g., agriculture and mining).

At the macro level, disease may result in a significant contraction in the production possibilities of an economy, perhaps even generating economic dislocation and decline in severe cases. Such contraction consequently imposes constraints on the revenues that the state may extract from the people through taxation, further limiting its capacity to deliver public services. Furthermore, multiple pathogens may interact through co-infection to augment the aggregate burden of disease on a population (e.g., malaria and HIV in sub-Saharan Africa). Severe epidemics may wither local, regional, and perhaps even macro-level domestic and regional economies.

Governance

Significant episodes of contagion may shift the dynamics of internal power away from society and toward the state, as the latter imposes draconian controls on the former in an attempt to limit the socio-economic disruption generated by the pathogen. Within society, disease-induced in-group/out-group psychological dynamics will often manifest as identity-based conflicts, generating or exacerbating competition and conflict between socio-economic classes and between elite factions and perhaps manifesting in the form of inter-ethnic conflict. Through the depletion of human capital assets and through declining tax revenues, contagion will induce a sclerotic effect within domestic institutions of governance, compromising the state's capacity to deliver essential services. As the institutions of governance become increasingly brittle and fragile, governments may exhibit increasing dysfunction and even paralysis.[4] Particularly severe outbreaks of infectious disease may undermine the legitimacy of pre-existing structures of hierarchy and authority within affected systems of governance. This may result in the de-legitimization of dominant societal institutions and religious entities, or the de-legitimization of the state itself in the face of its inability to provide required public goods and essential services.

Furthermore, as a result of the de-legitimization of existing structures of authority (including social and religious hierarchies), contagion may induce a breakdown of accepted behavioral norms, resulting in social chaos and generalized lawlessness. Criminal activity may increase, often dramatically, as the state's capacity to provide public goods, such as law and order, diminishes as a result of disease-induced declines in state capacity. The state, seeking to restore order, may often engage in severe (often draconian) measures to control the people, often provoking violent reactions and resulting in the further destabilization of the polity.

Ingenuity and Adaptation

Contagion often proves disruptive to societies, and it is extremely prob-lematic for governance, but it may result in the production of ingenuity that allows societies, economies, and structures of governance to switch to new modes of operation. For example, should the effects of the con-tagion fail to overwhelm the adaptive capacity of a polity, the shock may act as a catalyst and generate windows of opportunity for change. However, if the shock generated by contagion is too powerful it will exceed the endogenous adaptive capacity of the affected state, and con-sequently disease may shatter nations, as it did the majority of Amerin-dian cultures. Thus, the dynamic between contagion and ingenuity is revealed, reinforcing the claims of historians that disease has played an important role in determining the evolutionary trajectory of societies and states.

Effects at the International Level

Economic

Outbreaks of infectious disease (e.g., SARS) have the potential to induce the destabilization of regional economies, and to generate a drag on the productivity of the global economy. Outbreaks will typically impede the flow of trade goods from infected to uninfected regions, and such goods may be subject to quarantine or outright embargo. Such pathogen-induced impediments to the flow of goods and persons are exacerbated by fear and panic, which may be manipulated by domestic economic interest groups (as in the BSE affair) or by the global media. In certain cases (such as that of SARS) one may observe the complete embargo of possibly infected goods until the etiology of the pathogen, and its vectors of transmission, can be determined with some precision. Infectious disease may also undermine foreign investment in seriously affected regions because of perceptions of economic and political instability (e.g., HIV/AIDS), and fears that a firm's workers may succumb to the contagion, eroding the base of human capital within that firm. Thus, risk premiums will be significantly elevated in regions of significant pathogen prevalence. Collectively, this creates problems for global health governance as affected states have powerful disincentives to report outbreaks of disease to the WHO, or to accurately report the extent of the infection.

Governance
The balance of evidence suggests that contagion will *not* generate conflict between sovereign states, despite disease-induced shifts in relative power,[5] but may actually hasten an end to bellicose behavior. Relatively healthy countries will wisely avoid infected regions, insofar as armed conflict functions as a vector of disease transmission, increasing the probability of importing the pathogen in question to one's homeland through demobilization. Conversely, the evidence suggests that contagion has the capacity to breed political and economic acrimony between sovereign states but will not generate inter-state war. For example, negative outcomes in the domain of economics radiate as externalities to affect the domain of governance. As contagion obstructs international trade and commerce, it may induce political acrimony between affected states and/or regions, or between states and international organizations (as in the case of SARS).

Visitations of contagion expose persistent problems in cooperation between sovereign states and other agents in the realm of global health governance. Over time, differential levels in the aggregate burden of disease on populations may affect the relative power of those countries. Therefore, if a country A experiences serious burdens on population health resulting from the synchronous burden of malaria, onchocerciasis, and HIV/AIDS (for example) its economic productivity will be limited relative to a healthier country B over time. Disease will also likely compromise the infected country's institutional cohesion and efficacy, and the very capacity of the state to defend itself and to project power. Therefore, *ceteris paribus*, as a result of the heavy burden of disease on A, its aggregate power is diminished relative to B. Again, this does not seem to generate warfare between the parties in question, but it certainly may affect other political dimensions of country A's relationship with country B. For example, disease may reinforce existing structures of material inequities between countries. The burden of disease in tropical regions, due to pathogenic endemicity, reinforces the poverty of those affected countries, and traps them in a mutually reinforcing cycle of illness and poverty.

On Capacity, Power, and Legitimacy

As I have argued, the health of the population is central to economic productivity at the micro, sectoral, and macro levels, and the ingenuity (social and technical) that emanates from a healthy population drives innovation and adaptation. Thus, health generates prosperity,[6] and through processes of extraction (i.e., taxation) the state consequently derives its fiscal resources from this productive population base. Moreover, the state's investments in the health of its population confer additional legitimacy on the government, and those revenues extracted through taxation may subsequently be converted into public goods (such as education and law enforcement) that honor the social contract and further legitimize the state in the eyes of the people, stabilizing relations between state and society.

Furthermore, the state's economic resources are fungible and thus readily translated into military power. An expanding economy based on a healthy, productive, and innovative workforce thereby contributes directly to the martial and ideological power of the state over the longer term. In addition, a healthy pool of recruits is essential to maintaining the viability of any modern military, as is the health of a trained and highly skilled officer corps. In aggregate, then, the state's investments in the population's health contribute to socio-political cohesion and prosperity, which allow the state to maximize its material (and ideological) interests, to project power abroad, and to ensure its survival. The power and therefore the security of the state is, therefore, directly dependent on the health of its population. As Cicero noted centuries ago, political elites must recognize the wisdom of investing in the health and well-being of the body politic, in their own self-interest. Thus, investments in health create a virtuous spiral (or feedback loop) of increasing prosperity and socio-political stabilization.

Conversely, in the presence of epidemic levels of infection, with attendant debilitation and mortality, the productivity of workers will decline markedly. Poor health impairs cognitive function and consequently limits the production of ingenuity and the development of successful strategies of adaptation. Disease-induced stagnation and/or contraction of the economy and markets will then reduce the revenue streams available to the state through taxation, and correspondingly limit the capacity of the government to honor the social contract by delivering crucial public services. This will then negatively affect public perceptions of the government's legitimacy. Furthermore, as contagion erodes the human capital resources of affected bureaucracies, it will generate institutional fragility, sclerosis, and even paralysis. Over the longer term, as evident in the HIV/AIDS pandemic, the debilitation and/or mortality of enlisted ranks and of officers creates enormous problems in continuity for military institutions and for law enforcement. Therefore, disease undermines the coherence of the state and its ability to carry out its bureaucratic functions. The failure of the state to deliver public goods in a timely and effective manner will erode the perceived legitimacy of the regime in the eyes of the people.

Significant fear, anxiety, and even panic within a society may result in the stigmatization of the infected, or in the targeting of minority groups and campaigns of discrimination or violence directed toward them. Such psychological "constructions" may generate social instability, which the state perceives as a direct threat to its material interests, leading to governmental intervention (in draconian fashion). Paradoxically, such heavy-handed interventions by the government often trigger societal reactions against the state itself, occasionally manifesting in violence (riot and rebellion).

On Emergence and Non-Linear Change

The balance of the evidence suggests that epidemics and pandemics may exhibit emergent properties. Thus, emphasizing the connectivity between domains, the processes of violent conflict and inter-state warfare may interact with increasing speed of travel, increasing magnitude of trade, burgeoning population pools in mega-cities, and ecological degradation to facilitate the continuing emergence of zoonotic pathogens, and their endogenization within the human ecology. Therefore, we are likely to be confronted with many novel (and pathogenic) microbial agents in the centuries to come.[7]

Such complex and interactive processes of emergence contribute directly to the non-linear manifestations of pathogens as rapidly (often geometrically) expanding epidemics. While there is some preliminary evidence to suggest that certain domestic institutions of governance may respond to epidemic disease in non-linear fashion (i.e., rapid and punctuated change), such patterns of change are also observed at the international level.[8] Therefore, this domain of inquiry requires greater study before any firm conclusions may be drawn.

In the final analysis, emergence and proliferation of infectious agents should logically increase as processes of globalization accelerate. However, disease events will act as biotic countermeasures (negative feedback loops[9]) to slow the processes of globalization through reductions in the movement of trade goods and migrants, the depletion of human capital, and the erosion of economic productivity. In a very real sense, then, infectious disease acts as a negative feedback mechanism (or a natural brake) on the processes of globalization.

On reflection, punctuated-equilibrium theory appears to offer some utility in explaining the political outcomes associated with visitations of contagion. At the level of the sovereign state, the broad spectrum of political history clearly indicates that outbreaks of epidemic disease often resulted in rapid debilitation of military forces, in destabilization of relations between society and the state, and often in fractured or paralyzed domestic institutions of governance. In the most extreme cases, such as plague in Europe or smallpox in the Americas, pathogens resulted in the rapid and non-linear destabilization of entire polities as the contagion exceeded adaptive capacity. In the modern era, one can certainly argue, certain agents of contagion have contributed to the sclerosis and fragility of domestic institutions. For example, the pandemic influenza of 1918 certainly affected the prosecution of the war, as it directly undermined the German offensives in the spring and summer of 1918, undercut the economic productivity of affected polities, stressed Austrian institutions of governance, and even limited the efficacy of the American Expeditionary Forces in the latter months of the war.

The fracturing of domestic institutions is also evident in the case of BSE, wherein the emergence of prions generated rapid and profound institutional changes throughout British, French, and ultimately European structures of governance. The SARS epidemic also resulted in significant non-linear change in domestic structures of governance in affected polities, particularly Canada and China. Conversely, punctuated-equilibrium dynamics are not as apparent in the case of the HIV/AIDS pandemic, although arguably viral-induced stresses have directly contributed to the collapse of the Zimbabwean economy, imperiled the structural cohesion of the apparatus of governance, limited the state's provision of public goods, and propelled the state into its draconian repression of an increasingly disaffected and rebellious population. Indeed, this enduring consonance between the appearance of contagion and the hierarchical abuses of power by the state against its population is evidence of punctuated-equilibrium dynamics in operation, as the balance of power between society and the state is altered.

At the international level, the punctuated-equilibrium model is equally salient. The case studies illustrate that the 1918 influenza affected the balance of capabilities between the various protagonists in World War I. Further, contagion combined with war to generate stresses that contributed to the rapid demise of empires (German, Austrian, and Ottoman) in the fall of 1918. Thus, pandemic influenza altered the structure and trajectory of international relations in Europe in the decades that followed. Moreover, SARS resulted in the rapid (if ephemeral) empowerment of the World Health Organization relative to its sovereign member states, and BSE resulted in the rapid and permanent reform of various institutions within the construct of the European Union. Finally, the HIV/AIDS pandemic has resulted in the formation of a new division within the UN superstructure (UNAIDS) and has fomented the creation of a multilateral institution (the Global Fund for HIV, Tuberculosis and Malaria).

Epidemic disease often precipitates evolutionary change in affected societies and in the architecture of governance within an affected polity. Conversely, changes in technology, social relations, and ingenuity (technical and social) may stimulate corresponding evolutionary pressures within the microbial realm, accelerating prospects for mutation and the colonization of novel ecological niches. The interaction between human societies and microbes may, then, be seen as co-evolutionary in its dynamics, each side responding to changes in the other over time. Human societies do not simply adapt to some static exogenous environment; they change that microbial environment, leading to the decline of certain pathogens and the rise of new challengers.[10]

In the twentieth century, advances in public health and anti-microbials shifted the balance of power toward human societies. However, there is a significant difference in the velocity of change in each variable, as pathogens possess the capability of rapid genetic mutation, enhanced by the processes of swapping DNA between pathogens via surface antigens and transposons (antigenic shift). As pathogens acquire increased resistance through exposure to our anti-microbial armamentarium, the balance of power begins to shift back toward the microbes. Evidence of this is increasingly apparent in surging mortality from such resistant pathogens as methycillin-resistant staphylococcus aureus (MRSA), vancomycin-resistant enterococci (VRE), multi-drug resistant tuberculosis, and resistant strains of HIV and malaria. Furthermore, humanity's penchant for ecological degradation only increases the mathematical probability of emergence of novel (and perhaps lethal) pathogens from their natural reservoirs. Such dynamic systems are likely to exhibit oscillations in dominance between microbes and humans over considerable periods of time. Although we humans have enjoyed a recent period of dominance, the lack of significant progress in developing new anti-microbials suggests that the balance may be shifting to favor our microbial adversaries.

On Externalities

Health is a best perceived as a public good—that is, the health that I enjoy reduces the probability that infection may be transmitted from me (as host) to another human being and subsequently proliferate throughout the population. The concept of herd immunity stipulates that not all members of a population (say, of cattle) need be inoculated to provide the entire herd protection against a pathogenic agent. Specifically, only a certain majority of the herd need be inoculated such that the transmission rate of the pathogen is reduced to the extent that it cannot become a self-sustaining epidemic within the community of host organisms (rate <1). The same principle holds for human societies, as the health of my neighbor acts as a public good to enhance my health by limiting the probability of disease transmission throughout the community at large. Health is therefore both non-rivalrous and non-exclusive, and the good health of individuals in a community generates a collective or public good experienced by the polity in question, and perhaps the entire human species.

Conversely, the proliferation of contagion generates externalities, or "public bads,"[11] that impose diffuse and pernicious costs on others in society, and perhaps throughout the global system. Within a society, infected hosts act as vectors for the distribution of a pathogen (or pathogens), inadvertently visiting empirical harm on others. The negative impacts of illness function as externalities, imposing a significant range of costs on the larger society—including health-care costs, rising insurance premiums, the destruction of the endogenous base of human capital (so evident in the HIV/AIDS pandemic), and diminished economic productivity. Furthermore, at the international level, countries that are impoverished and/or destabilized as a result of contagion may consequently generate externalities that affect other countries, other regions, or the international system. For example, the initial failure of China to contain the SARS epidemic resulted in the proliferation of the disease in Southeast Asia and North America, generating significant economic costs to the entire Pacific Rim region. Similarly, the policies of denial and obfuscation by leaders in Zimbabwe and South Africa regarding HIV/AIDS have directly facilitated the prevalence of the pathogen throughout the region,[12] and such entrenchment of the virus in Southern Africa now functions as a mechanism to distribute the pathogen on a global scale.

Implications for Political Theory

I have employed a republican revision of the Realist paradigm which holds that certain manifestations of epidemic disease present a distinct threat to the material interests of the sovereign state. This threat is generated through the disease-induced destruction and debilitation of the population, the erosion of productivity and prosperity, fear-induced social destabilization, the disruption of institutions of governance, and the consequent erosion of the state's power relative to unaffected rivals in the international system.

A caveat, however: orthodox Realist responses that advocate strategies of self-help in an increasingly globalized world are problematic for states with low endogenous capacity.[13] Indeed, even the United States, with its high capacity, had great difficulty containing just one individual who was infected with a highly resistant form of tuberculosis in the spring of 2007. Complex interdependence, a facet of Liberalism, must thus also be imported into republican security theory. Ethnocentric visions of global health that exclusively advocate self-help, to the exclusion of building capacity in the developing countries, are myopic and likely to be ineffective in the global containment of emergent pathogens (e.g., a novel lethal influenza). Republican security theory is therefore a useful analytical lens through which to view the *threat* posed by contagion; however, the development of endogenous capacity for containment must be supplemented by cooperative international initiatives, as the *means* by which to effectively maintain surveillance and containment of pathogens on a global scale.[14] Such cooperation is essential to the protection of the material interests of all states. Furthermore, a republican variant of Realist theory allows for interactivity between the domestic and systems level of analysis, such that problems at the domestic level may generate externalities that destabilize the international system.

Recommendations

The best way to curtail future epidemics (and pandemics) is to augment the endogenous capacity of health-care infrastructure and to improve the basal health of populations, particularly throughout the developing countries. Such investments are logical because the fundamental conditions for disease emergence are accelerating as a result of the processes of globalization (increased population density, ecological degradation, rapid transportation technologies, and mass migration), yet in many developing areas disease surveillance and containment capacity is low or nonexistent.

Given that global public health can be understood as a public good, the costs of providing such goods (epidemiological surveillance and containment) should be borne by the international community, although continued diplomatic leadership by a hegemonic coalition of states will doubtless remain central. Further, developed countries should possess (or develop) a level of "surge capacity" to deal with epidemic events that generate mass morbidity and mortality, such as a new lethal pandemic influenza. At present there is little surge capacity within the United States as a result of its uniquely market-driven health-care system. Indeed, there are not enough beds, respirators, and nurses in the United States to effectively deal with a flu pandemic on the level of 1918. The presence of weak and often dysfunctional international institutions that are chronically lacking in funding (the WHO), and which occasionally suffer from politicized and/or weak leadership, complicates proactive responses. While the recently revised International Health Regulations should assist in increasing global response capacity to pathogenic threats,[15] the regime continues to lack any substantive capacity to enforce compliance by its member states. Thus, it is incumbent upon states to lead the way in assembling regional coalitions to deal with emergent health threats.

What further measures should be taken to bring the concept of "health security" into the mainstream of security studies?

Reduce Ethnocentrism   Orthodox security analysts remain wedded to the concept that the developing countries are essentially non-strategic, unless petroleum reserves (or terrorists) exist in that region. The prevailing security literature must change to integrate the concerns of developing countries. Moreover, the literature is also guilty of exceptional anthropocentrism, regarding threats to security as resulting exclusively from human agency. As Hurricane Katrina demonstrated, natural processes and events can also generate profound disruptions to the prosperity, coherence, effective governance, legitimacy, and security of sovereign states. The destruction visited on modern societies by the 1918 influenza pandemic and by the modern manifestation of HIV argues for increasingly ecocentric and non-ethnocentric perspectives within the security literature.

Encourage Scientific Literacy   As Deudney argues, much of the current political science literature completely disregards those material-contextual factors that have influenced societies and states over millennia. In this era of faddish post-modernism, such filters of abstraction have grown so pronounced that some social scientists now question the empirical existence of pathogens. Simply put, many political scientists are uncomfortable in the realm of the hard sciences, and very few have any significant understanding of microbiology, epidemiology, or medicine. Thus, the education of social scientists in the core concepts of biology, ecology, and public health will provide for greater comprehension of the risks involved in pathogenic emergence and proliferation. Conversely, those in public health and medicine would do well to become conversant in the tenets of political science, so as to understand the vagaries of the political process.

Counter Threat Myopia   The terrorist attacks of 2001, and the subsequent wars in Afghanistan and Iraq have deflected the security community's attention away from those infectious disease threats which had been on the radar at the United Nations Security Council in the spring of 2001. The prevailing obsession with anthropocentric threats (i.e., terrorism) leaves little cognitive space for scholars or policy makers to be concerned about subtle and attenuated threats, and makes it difficult to observe health and environmental challenges to security.

Increase Historical Literacy   In recent years, the discipline of political science (particularly the American school) has bowed to the quantitative orthodoxy of econometrics, and to the dogma of parsimony and linearity. In complex and non-linear systems (such as the interactions between pathogens, economies, states, and societies), an exclusive focus on parsimonious empirical methods may be misleading.[16] Many newly minted PhDs in political science may be able to run advanced multi-variate regressions but have never read the canon of republican political thought embodied in the work of Aristotle, Plato, Thucydides, Machiavelli, Hobbes, Montesquieu and Rousseau. Beyond the historical community, academia is largely unaware of the historical relations between health, governance, and power. In order to acquire a more balanced perspective, political scientists might study more history and anthropology, and less econometrics.

Provision of Evidence   As the frequency of catastrophic epidemics has declined, evidence of the malign effects of contagion on state cohesion, power, and security has been relegated to the past (as is true of pandemic influenza) or has been largely dismissed as a scourge of the developing countries. Thus, scholars must be vigilant both in their investigation of the relations between such variables and in their attempts to remind the current generation of our continuing vulnerability to emergent pathogens. As the epidemiologist Stephen Morse reminds us, there is always a novel pathogen in the pipeline of nature.[17] To that end, a deeper and cross-national investigation into the effects of the pandemic influenza of 1918 on prosperity, governance, and security should be conducted posthaste. Further cross-national investigations into the effects of the current HIV/AIDS pandemic on governance should also be undertaken.

Acknowledge Cognitive Limitations   Humans have been programmed biologically to respond to imminent threats, such as a proximate predator. Therefore, they are far more likely to perceive temporally proximate "events" as related to significant threats, as opposed to attenuated and often difficult to observe "processes" such as ecological destruction and the gradual winnowing of a population by consecutive waves of contagion. The environment-and-security debate has been witness to similar issues of societal Attention Deficit Disorder, as few pay attention to the attenuated processes of ozone depletion (or global climate change) until the system reaches a critical threshold, whereupon the issue "suddenly" becomes a profound threat to the human species and to the security of sovereign states. Threats to global health often exhibit similar properties, particularly stealth pathogens such as HIV/AIDS.

While the human species has significantly reduced its vulnerability to contagion over the centuries, this reduction in vulnerability is primarily pathogen-specific. Certain microbial agents (such as pandemic influenza) still represent an enormous threat to the national security of all polities. Profound variance in the capacity of states and in the attributes of populations suggests that different countries will be vulnerable to different pathogens. Thus, one pathogen (e.g., HIV/AIDS) may combine with others to generate a profound burden of disease that threatens the prosperity, stability, and security of a certain country (e.g., Zimbabwe). The same pathogens may not threaten a developed country such as Canada, which instead proved quite vulnerable to the SARS coronavirus. Thus, pathogenic threats to security are highly contextual. Despite technological optimism and anthropocentrism, human societies remain firmly ensconced within the ecological constraints of the natural world, and will remain vulnerable to the continuing processes of pathogen emergence in the centuries to come. Therefore, it would be expedient to accelerate our efforts in improving global population health, and in developing a global infrastructure for the effective surveillance and containment of contagion.

On a positive note, the extreme destabilization witnessed during historical plagues and pestilences has diminished greatly over the centuries. Advances in technical ingenuity have resulted in the development of antimicrobial agents, and in improved nutrition for much of the world's population. Social ingenuity has also improved over the centuries as the architecture of global health governance has begun to improve, and as national governments now comprehend that excessively draconian (contagionist) policies can spawn and exacerbate existing conflicts between societal factions (or classes) and the state itself. Certain contagionist policies remain in place (such as the necessity for quarantine and social distancing). However, certain polities have become increasingly draconian in the face of contagion, notably China (SARS) and Zimbabwe (HIV).

On a cautionary note, despite humanity's recent advances in the domain of public health, there is reason to be concerned about the proliferation of resistant infections which diminish the efficacy of our existing anti-microbial armamentarium. Furthermore, pharmaceutical companies often eschew investments in new classes of anti-microbial prophylaxis, claiming that the returns on investment are insufficient. Thus, many of the diseases of the developing countries (e.g., malaria) continue to proliferate because the people they affect are unable to pay exorbitant prices for new classes of medication. The scale and velocity of ecological degradation is troubling, in that disruptions to biological equilibria may generate new niches for pathogenic emergence or mutation. Global climate change is particularly troubling, as it will lead to the latitudinal and altitudinal expansion of vectors (e.g., mosquitoes), permitting the proliferation of various infective agents (e.g., malaria) in human populations that possess no genetic or acquired immunity to the pathogen. In the case of malaria, increasing temperatures will also increase the biting rate of the vectors, and even the incubation rate of the plasmodium itself, intensifying the burden of disease on affected populations. It is certainly reasonable to suspect that climate change may also result in the emergence of novel pathogenic agents that may thrive in warmer and wetter environments.

The centrality of *physis* to republican political thought facilitates the location of pathogenic threats to national security within the domain of the wider "environmental security" discourse. As human actions continue to generate significant disturbances within the ecosystems of the planet, such deviations facilitate the emergence of novel pathogens and the mutation of existing strains. The hubris of the human species, the ascendance of the ideational and the ignorance of the material, and the illusion that humanity has been liberated from the constraints of the natural world are problematic. The human species must recognize its place within the complex web of life, eschew anthropocentric orthodoxy in favor of ecocentric perspectives, and return a modicum of equilibrium to the biosphere. The development of ecological consciousness (and praxis) in societies and markets, will permit a return to greater biotic equilibrium, reducing the speed of pathogenic emergence and mutation. Through such tactics, humanity may diminish its vulnerability to contagion, and to the chaos it may generate.

Notes

Introduction

1. Schumpeter 2005.

2. On punctuated equilibria, see Gould 2002, pp. 765–768.

3. McNeill 1977; Crosby 1986, 2003a,b.

4. Notwithstanding the valuable contributions of those few scholars involved in the environment-and-security debate, such as Dennis Pirages, Richard Matthew, Ken Conca, Kent Butts, Miranda Schreurs, Thomas Homer-Dixon, Marc Levy, Colin Kahl, Geoffrey Dabelko, and Nils Petter Gleditsch.

5. Deudney 2006, p. xii.

6. Braudel (1993, p. 338) notes the pernicious effect of the Black Death on early European societies: "From the tenth to the thirteenth century. . . . Europe was active, full of life, and expanding rapidly. Then came the Black Death and a brutal, catastrophic decline. Everything suffered, even the progress of Christianity, during the long series of disturbances and strife that historians call the Hundred Years' War (1337–1453)."

7. Such issues will be discussed in greater detail in chapter 6.

8. Consilience is defined as the jumping together of knowledge across disciplinary boundaries. See Wilson 1998 and Whewell 1840. Whewell, who coined the term, wrote: "The Consilience of Inductions takes place when an Induction, obtained from one class of facts, coincides with an Induction, obtained from another different class. This Consilience is a test of the truth of the Theory in which it occurs."

9. On processes and dynamics of globalization, see Krugman and Venables 1995; Stiglitz 2006; O'Rourke and Williamson 2001; Bhagwati 2004.

10. Davis and Kimball 2001.

11. See McMichael 2003; Price-Smith 2002; Epstein 2000, 2001.

12. Elbe 2002; Ostergard 2002.

13. See Poku 2002; Farmer 2003.

14. Thucydides 1980, pp. 400–408.

15. McNeill 1977, p. 134. See also Verity et al. 1999, pp. 213–220.

16. Crosby 1986.

17. Severe Acute Respiratory Syndrome.

18. Rosen 2007, p.173.

19. Pirages 1995.

Chapter 1

1. Kuhn 1962, pp. 17–18.

2. Rousseau 1968, p. 130.

3. Ibid., p. 77.

4. Thomas Hobbes is also viewed as a central figure in republican (and, by extension, Classical Realist) thought. See Hobbes 1985.

5. Deudney 2006, p. 6.

6. Ibid., p. 13.

7. See Kelly 1990, pp. 14–34.

8. See Aristotle 1984. Also see the summary of this debate in Onuf 1998.

9. See Plato, *The Laws*, 676b–682e; Plato, *Timaeus*, 23b.

10. See Deudney's terminology (2006, p. 95).

11. Plato, *The Laws*; Plato, *Timaeus*; Aristotle, *Politics*; Thucydides, *History of the Peloponnesian War*; Machiavelli, *The Prince* and *The Discourses*; Montesquieu, *Spirit of the Laws*; Rousseau, *The Social Contract*; Hobbes, *Leviathan*.

12. See Glacken 1967.

13. Montesquieu, *Spirit of the Laws*, book 19, section 14, p. 299.

14. Deudney 2006, pp. 117–118.

15. See, e.g., Homer-Dixon 1999; Deudney and Matthew 1999; Price-Smith 2002a.

16. Deudney 2006, p. 17.

17. Strauss 1953, p. 81.

18. Waltz 1990; van Evera 2001; Mearshimer 2003; Buzan and Little 2000.

19. See, e.g., Wendt 1999.

20. Onuf 1998, p. 20.

21. Rosenau 1997, p. 3.

22. For a lengthy discussion of the relationship between health and state capacity, see Price-Smith 2002a.

23. Thucydides 1980, pp. 400–408.

24. Note that the vicissitudes of human nature and their effects upon policy decision making are discussed at length throughout the republican literature. Early-to-mid-twentieth-century Realism (until the 1970s) maintained this focus on human nature. See in particular Waltz 1954 and the various works of Hans Morgenthau.

25. Putnam 2000, pp. 20–26.

26. Social complexity may range from those early hunter-gatherer societies that exhibited low levels of complexity to the exceedingly complex social networks of modern societies such as Germany, Canada, the United States, or Japan. According to the archaeologist Joseph Tainter (1988, p. 23), the term 'complexity' "is generally understood to refer to such things as the size of a society, the number and distinctiveness of its parts, the variety of specialized roles that it incorporates, the number of distinct social personalities present, and the variety of mechanisms for organizing these into a coherent, functioning whole."

27. Economic productivity declines as a direct result of the morbidity and mortality induced by the pathogen in question. (Hence the interactivity between the demographic and economic domains).

28. Price-Smith 2001, pp. 1–14.

29. Migdal 1988, p. 35.

30. Ibid., p. 19. On Weberian conceptions of the state, see Rheinstein 1954, p. 342. See also Weber 1964, p. 156.

31. State autonomy from societal factions is seen as a central component of its capacity, as defined in the writings of Stephen Krasner and Peter Katzenstein. See, in particular, Krasner 1978 and Katzenstein 1978.

32. Adapted from pp. 25–26 of Price-Smith 2002.

33. McNeill 1976, p. 2.

34. Price-Smith 2002a, pp. 30–39.

35. Peterson and Shellman 2006, pp. 1–3.

36. Proponents of qualitative research include Colin Kahl (2006) and Thomas Homer-Dixon (1999).

37. Kuhn 1970, p. 15.

38. Jervis 1997, p. 43.

39. Rosenberg 1966, p. 453.

40. Walt 1996, p. 177.

41. Significant proponents of process tracing include Thomas Homer-Dixon (1999) and Alexander George (1979).

42. See Sprout and Sprout 1968, p. 55.

43. Phillips 1976, p. 14.

44. Jervis 1997, p. 5.

45. Ibid., p. 6. For other accounts of complex systems from international relations theory, see Bull 1977, pp. 8–16; Waltz 1979, p. 79; Gilpin 1981; Hoffman 1961, pp. 207–208.

46. McNeill 1989, pp. 1–2.

47. McMichael 2001; Price-Smith 2002a; Aron and Patz 2001.

48. Jervis 1997, p. 28.

49. Price-Smith 2001.

50. Aristotle, *Physics*, II v (197a11–13), in Aristotle 1984, volume I, p. 336.

51. On non-linear effects within the social sciences, see Kiel and Elliot 1966; Brown 1995; Beyerchen 1992–93.

52. Campbell led the SARS Commission's Inquiry into the processes of breakdown in Ontario's public health structures during the SARS epidemic of spring 2003.

53. Durkheim 1938, p. xlvii. See also Anderson 1972.

54. See also Laughlin 2005.

55. Bartlett 1960.

56. Morse 1993; Lederberg 1997.

57. Jervis 1997, p. 39.

58. For the seminal "functionalist" model, see Haas 1964.

59. On the pervasive destruction of Amerindian societies and institutions of governance via smallpox, see Fenn 2004.

60. Krasner 1984.

61. North 1990.

62. Baumgartner and Jones 2002.

63. See Speth and Repetto 2006; Romanelli and Tushman 1994; Breunig and Koski 2006.

64. Blyth 2002.

65. Rosenau 1997, pp. 11, 17.

66. Ibid., pp. 16, 21.

67. Diehl and Goertz 2000.

68. The balance of epidemiological and historical evidence indicates that *Yersinia pestis* was indeed exogenous to Europe, and that it was a zoonosis emanating from rodent reservoirs in Central Asia.

69. On the role of ingenuity in political adaptation, see Homer-Dixon 2000.

70. Watts 2003, p. 4.

71. Ibid., p. 96.

72. Slack 1992, p. 8.

73. Deudney 2006, pp. 32–33.

74. Jervis 1970. See also Cottam and Cottam 2001; Herrmann et al. 1997.

75. Thagard and Kroon 2006; Marcus et al. 2000; Morris et al. 2003; Lodge and Taber 2005.

76. Posner 2004, p. 168.

77. Ibid., p. 169.

78. Sunstein 2002, p. 61.

Chapter 2

1. Cicero, *De Legibus*, Book III, Part III, Sub. VIII.

2. See, e.g., Baldwin 2005. See also Diamond 1999.

3. Among them are Dennis Pirages, Andrew Price-Smith, Robert Ostergard, and Stefan Elbe.

4. The material evidence of polio infection manifested in the form of distinct lesions on the bones of the infected individual. On polio, see Wells 1964. On tuberculosis, see Formicola et al. 1987; Mercer 1964; Evans 1998.

5. See Steinbock 1976; Baker and Armelagos 1988; El-Najjar 1979; Moller-Christensen 1969.

6. Consilience may be defined as the jumping together of knowledge across disciplinary boundaries. It does not necessarily imply the search for meta-theory, but rather the pursuit of interdisciplinary knowledge. See Wilson 1999.

7. Gaddis 1997, p. 75.

8. Harvey Mansfield, as quoted in Jennifer Howard, "In Jefferson Lecture, Harvey Mansfield reflects on what the humanities can teach science and political science," *Chronicle of Higher Education*, May 9, 2007.

9. See Procopius 1914, volume I, pp. 450–455.

10. See Galen 1821–1833, volume 7, pp. 287–294. See also Galen 1969.

11. Hippocrates 1923.

12. Thucydides 1980, p. 155.

13. Niccolo Machiavelli, *Description of the Plague at Florence in 1527*, as quoted in on pp. 216–217 of Nohl 2006.

14. Zinsser 1934, p. 128.

15. Ibid., p. 129.

16. Hence the name of Zinsser's classic treatise, *Rats, Lice and History*.

17. Historically, the term 'plague' has been applied to any form of epidemic or pandemic disease, and not specifically to the bacteria *Yersinia pestis* which actually generates bubonic plague.

18. See Durack and Littman, as cited in University of Maryland Medical Center, "Plague of Athens" (press release, January 1999; http://www.umm.edu).

19. Such investigations were conducted using DNA samples of dental pulp from exhumed cadavers of those who died during this period.

20. Papagrigorakis et al. 2006.

21. Thucydides 1980, p. 155.

22. Longrigg 1992, pp. 21, 43. See also the account of Diodorus, cited on p. 11 of Prinzing 1916.

23. Gomme 1981, pp. 1–5. See also Gomme 1967, p. 6.

24. McNeill 1977, p. 94.

25. Longrigg 1992, p. 32.

26. See Durack and Littman, as cited in University of Maryland Medical Center, "Plague of Athens" (press release, January 1999; http://www.umm.edu).

27. McNeill 1977, p. 126.

28. Alternative origins for the pathogen include Eastern Africa. According to the observations of Evagrius Scholasticus (1846), the pestilence originated in Ethiopia. William Rosen (2007, p. 220) supports this alternative hypothesis.

29. McNeill 1977, pp. 101–106. See also Biraben and Le Goff 1969.

30. Russell 1968.

31. Rosen 2007, p. 3.

32. See Procopius 1917, 23:1.

33. Procopius, as cited on p. 146 of Zinsser 1934.

34. Gibbon, as quoted on pp. 147–148 of Zinsser 1934.

35. Russell 1968.

36. Allen 1979.

37. See Findlay and Lundahl 2006.

38. Dols 1977, pp 17–18.

39. McNeill 1977, p. 113, Zinsser 1934, p. 133, Rosen 2007, pp. 321–324.

40. McNeill 1977, p. 121.

41. On how it affected the Mamluk Empire, which ranged from Egypt to Syria during the initial phase of the contagion, see Dols 1977, p. 143.

42. Foster 1976.

43. Recent findings by the historian Christopher Dyer (2002, p. 215) suggest that mortality may have approached 50 percent across Europe.

44. Hatcher 1977, p. 25.

45. Slack 1992, p. 4. See also Slack 1985.

46. Dols 1977, pp. 168–174, 183.

47. Watts 1997, p. 26; Dols 1977, p. 162; Irwin 1986, p. 141.

48. Abu-Lughod 1971, p. 38.

49. Dols 1977, p. 282.

50. Ayalon 1946, pp. 67–73.

51. McNeill 1977, p. 150.

52. Ibid., p. 162.

53. Watts 1997, pp. 20–21.

54. Nohl 2006, p. 164.

55. Ambroise Pare, as cited on p. 167 of Nohl 2006.

56. Nohl 2006, p. 111.

57. Slack 1992, p. 4.

58. Shatzmiller 1974; Kelly 138–140, 153.

59. Slack 1992, p. 16.

60. Nohl 2006, p. 182.

61. Such legislation stipulated that Jewish populations were to be barred from residency in Strasbourg for two centuries (Nohl 2006, p. 184).

62. Nohl 2006, p. 185.

63. Ibid., p. 176.

64. Kelly 2005, p. 267.

65. Chandavarkar 1992.

66. Ibid., pp. 232–233.

67. See Campbell 1931, p. 162. See also Wood 1792–1796, volume 1, p. 449.

68. See Oestrich 1982; Cook 1989.

69. Rosen 1993, p. 44.

70. Slack 1992, p. 15; Rosen 1993, p. 45.

71. Watts 1997, p. 23. See also Biraben 1976, pp. 86–90.

72. Watts 1997, p. 21.

73. Cipolla 1977, p. 13.

74. Watts 1997, p. 24. See also Kamen 1980, pp. 50–53.

75. Watts 1997, p. 25. See also Rothenberg 1973, p. 19; Jelavich 1983, pp. 144–148.

76. See McNeill 1976.

77. Such arguments are made in greater detail in Price-Smith 2002a.

78. Chandavarkar 1992, p. 204.

79. Ibid., pp. 207–208.

80. Ibid., p. 210.

81. See Ruffer 1921, pp. 166–178; Oldstone 1998, p. 28. See also Hopkins 1983.

82. Tucker 2001, p.7.

83. Hopkins 2002, p. 22.

84. Zinsser 1934, p. 137.

85. Hopkins 2002, p. 34.

86. Ibid., pp. 37, 41; Glyn and Glyn 2004, p. 1.

87. Hopkins 2002, p. 44.

88. Oldstone 1998, pp. 3, 33. See also Hopkins 1983.

89. Tucker 2001, pp. 9–10.

90. Crosby 1986, p. 200. See also Denevan 1976.

91. Thornton 1987, pp. 36, 90.

92. Dobyns 1966, pp. 395–416.

93. McNeill 1977, pp. 180–181.

94. Ibid., p. 190.

95. See Lockhart 1992, pp. 112–116; Gruzinski 1993, p. 81.

96. Watts 1997, p. 91.

97. Ibid., p. 90. See also Lovell 1992.

98. McNeill 1977, p. 183.

99. Fenn 2001, pp. 62–67.

100. Both Hegel and Clausewitz would appear to have died during the cholera outbreak of 1831, which ravaged Prussia.

101. Poznansky 1996.

102. Watts 1997, p. 167.

103. Thus, cholera mortality data are likely prone to significant underestimate.

104. For more on the shortcomings of pre-1884 cholera data, see Watts 1997, pp. 172–173.

105. Evans 1992, p. 154. See also McGrew 1965, p. 3.

106. Delaporte 1986, p. 50.

107. Ibid., p. 53.

108. Snowdon 1995, p. 149.

109. Evans 1992, p.158.

110. McGrew 1965, pp. 106–107.

111. Hays 2003, p. 138.

112. Watts 1997, p. 192.

113. Durey 1979, p. 157.

114. Evans 1992, p. 159.

115. Watts 1997, pp, 192–194.

116. Ibid., p. 196.

117. Calcott 1984, p. 75.

118. Markel 1993.

119. Hays 2003, pp. 140–141. See also Sigerist 1962, p. 80.

120. Anker and Schaaf 2000, p. 11.

121. Ibid., p. 107.

122. Alexander Hamilton, as quoted on p. 107 of Powell 1993.

123. George Washington, as quoted on p. 108 of Powell 1993.

124. Powell 1993, p. 65.

125. Ibid., p. 68.

126. Ibid., p. 109.

127. Watts 1997, p. 243.

128. Ibid., p. 244.

129. Ibid., p. 244.

130. Ibid., p. 245. See also Bloom 1993, pp. 230–231; Baker 1968.

131. Watts 2003, p. 104.

132. The Galenic tradition held that disease was primarily the result of "environmental" factors such as bad airs or malign waters, or that disease was generated by poverty.

133. In this sense, the persistent ineptitude of the epistemic community of physicians led to severe declines in their perceived legitimacy by political elites. Thus, the contagionists rose to power as a rival epistemic community, albeit a rather severe one. On the concept of rivalry between epistemic communities in the domain of health and policy, see Youde 2007.

134. Watts 2003, p. 104.

135. See Rosen 1993, p. 81.

136. See Rousseau 2005.

137. On the distinction between social and technical ingenuity, see Homer-Dixon 2000.

138. Indeed, the history of polemics between these two rival epistemic communities often prevents any sober and analytical discussion between the two camps.

139. Baldwin 2005, p. 93.

140. Watts 2003, p. 104.

141. Baldwin 2005, p. 72.

142. Evans 1992, p. 163. See also Luckin 1984.

143. Evans 1992, p. 163–4.

144. Baldwin 2005, p. 52.

145. Ibid., p. 66.

146. In recent years, the literature has begun to refer to those who recognize the association between health and issues of national security as *securitizers* and to

those who oppose such relations as *anti-securitizers*. Such terminology is inappropriate and demonstrates a profoundly shallow understanding of the historical and theoretical antecedents, suggesting that the former camp is seeking to impose a new ideology of security on the domain of public health. Given that contagionist thought originated in northern Italy, and that the practices of those in Firenza were emulated across Europe, it is appropriate to refer to this school as the Firenza or Florentine school. Those who have adopted the contrasting position, holding that disease was not in fact contagious, but rather environmental and induced by poverty, I shall dub the Galenic school.

Chapter 3

1. There are many excellent historical accounts of World War I and its aftermath. See, e.g., Keegan 2000; Macmillan 2003; Chickering 2004; Hermann 1997; Ferguson 2000.

2. Byerly 2005, p. 4.

3. Noymer and Garenne 2003; Zinsser 1934.

4. Crosby 2003a, p. 323.

5. See Frost 1918.

6. Sydenstricker 1918.

7. Crosby 2003a, p. 205.

8. Rice and Palmer 1993, p. 394.

9. Brown 1987.

10. Great Britain, House of Commons, Accounts and Papers, Session February 10, 1920, volume 32, Colonial Reports—Annual, no. 1032, Sierra Leone.

11. Patterson 1983.

12. Rice 1983.

13. Mills 1986.

14. Samoan Epidemic Commission Report, New Zealand House of Representatives, Appendices to the Journals (1919), H-31C, pp 1–11.

15. Taubenberger and Morens 2006, p. 15. See also Johnson and Mueller 2002, p. 105.

16. Johnson and Mueller 2002, pp. 105–115.

17. Taubenberger 1999.

18. Byerly 2005, p. 92.

19. Preliminary research by Canada's National Microbiology Laboratory now supports the hypothesis that the flu generated a cytokinetic storm, that drove the immune systems of hosts to overreact and destroy healthy tissues, frequently leading to death. See Helen Branswell, "Spanish Flu study finds why it was so virulent," *Globe and Mail*, Toronto, January 18, 2007.

20. *Statistisches Jahrbuch für das Deutsche Reich 1924/25* (Berlin, 1925), pp. 44–49.

21. Ghobarah et al. (2003) note that the negative health effects of war often persist for years beyond the cessation of hostilities.

22. See Crosby 2003a, p. 15. See also Phillips and Killingray 2003, pp. 5–6. Recently this view has been challenged by the British virologist John Oxford, who posits that the virus first emerged among young British troops based at Etaples, in northern France, during the winter of 1917. See Oxford et al. 2005.

23. Ewald 1994, pp. 110–111.

24. Ibid., p. 112.

25. Byerly 2005, p. 11.

26. Author's interview with Dr. Wilfried Witte, Berlin, August 7, 2006.

27. Johnson and Mueller 2002, p. 105.

28. Byerly 2005, p. 183.

29. Ibid., p. 187. See also US Congress, Senate, Senate Doc 40, Battle Deaths in the Great War, June 23, 1919, 66th Congress, 1st session.

30. Ayres 1919, p. 123.

31. Church 1921, p. 384; Bainbridge 1921, p. 384.

32. *War Department Annual Record*, 1919, pp. 2749–2751.

33. See Ayres 1919, p. 127.

34. Quoted on p. 104 of Byerly 2005.

35. Seidule 1997, p. 259.

36. Crosby 2003a, p. 127.

37. Ibid., p. 49.

38. Ibid., p. 62; Coffman 1987, pp. 82–83.

39. Byerly 2005, p. 107.

40. *War Dept Annual Report, 1919*, volume 1, part III, p. 3237.

41. Crosby 2003a, p. 155; *Eighty-Eighth Division in the World War, 1914–1918* (Syncope Whaleback Crawford, 1919), pp. 15–16, 108.

42. Quoted in Byerly 2005, p. 108.

43. Byerly 2005, p. 6.; Ayres 1919), pp. 125–126; *Medical Department in the World War*, volume 9 (Washington, 1920), pp. 66–69.

44. Ayres 1919, p. 123.

45. See Ayres 1919, p. 124.

46. Crosby 2003a, p. 122.; *Annual Reports of the Navy Department* 1919, p. 2439.

47. Crosby 2003a, p. 205.

48. Charles Lynch, Authoritative Data of the Medical Department. Records of the Surgeon General of the Army, Entry 29, Box 159, National Archives and Records Administration.

49. *Medical Department in the World War*, volume 9, pp. 66–67.

50. War Department, *Annual Reports*, 1919, volume 1, part II, pp. 1429–41.

51. Ibid., pp. 1437, 2012.

52. Byerly 2005, p. 99.

53. Tomkins 1992, p. 441.

54. Hundredth 1991, p. 278.

55. Crosby 2003a, p. 153.

56. See Niall Johnson, 1918–1919 Influenza Pandemic Mortality in England and Wales, Table XX of Supplement to the Eighty-First Annual Report to the Registrar General, London, UK (1920), www.adhs.ac.uk.

57. Oldstone 1998, p. 173. See also Livesey 1989.

58. Bessel 1993, p. 46.

59. See Beauftragter des Bayer. Kreigsministeriums beim Preuss. Kreigsamt vom den Staatskommisar für die Demobilmachung, Berlin, 16 Nov. 1918, Abt. IV, MKr 14412.

60. Crosby 2003a, p. 160.

61. Ludendorff 1919, volume 2, p. 227.

62. As cited on p. 195 of Volkmann 1925.

63. Crosby 2003a, p. 27.

64. *Der Sanitatsdienst im Gefechts- und Schlachtenverlauf im Weltkriege 1914/1918* (Mittler & Sohn, 1938), p. 121.

65. See Garrison 1920, p. 437.

66. Bessel 1993, p. 224. See also Thuringisches Statistiches Landesamt, *Statistisches Handbuch für das Land Thuringen*, 1922 (Weimar, 1922), p. 62; Statistisches Amt, *Statistsches Jarhbuch der Stadt Leipzig*, v, 1915–1918 (Leipzig, 1921), pp. 50–51, 61.

67. Ibid. and *Statistiches Jahrbuch für das Deutsche Reich 1927* (Berlin, 1927); Statistiches Reichsamt, Statistik des Deutschen Reichs, cccxvi: *Die Bewegung der Bevolkerung in den Jahren 1922 und 1923 und die Uhrsachen der Sterbefalle in den Jahren 1920 bis 1923* (Berlin, 1926), pp. 60–63.

68. See GStAM, Rep. 120, BB, Abt. VII, Fach 1, no. 30, Band 2, fos. 121–2: Oberpräsident der Provinz Shlesein vom Ministerium für Handel und Gewerbe, Breslau, 22 Dec 1918.

69. Bessel 1993, p. 149.

70. Ibid., pp. 39, 126.

71. Oxford et al. (2002, 2005) suggest that the first such epidemic manifestation of a novel and lethal strain of influenza may have emerged in the British forces at Etaples, France in 1916. Such British origins might account for the diminished morbidity and mortality observed in British forces.

72. Regarding the relationship between influenza and pneumonia: There is a robust record of influenza creating the preconditions for secondary infection by pneumonia. Another possible explanation is that physicians in 1918 had a difficult time in identifying the illness, and may have inadvertently classified a death from influenza as a death from pneumonia. Regardless, the body count remains significant, particularly as much of the mortality was significantly under-reported.

73. See Farwell 1999; Keene 2001; Zeigler 2000.

74. *New York Times*, October 20, 1918.

75. Crosby 2003a, p. 207.

76. Ibid., p. 75.

77. Ibid., p. 75.

78. Ibid., p. 76.

79. Ibid., p. 98.

80. Ibid., p. 81.

81. Ibid., p. 95.

82. See Schafer et al. 1993.

83. Monto 2005.

84. Ghendon 1994.

85. Safranek 1991.

86. See Dutton 1988; Silverstein 1981.

87. Li et al. 2004.

88. The pathogen exhibits significant variation in lethality based on cluster and region, but a mortality rate greater than 30 percent is typically observed in infected patients. See Kaye and Pringle 2003. Accurate assessments are hampered by enormous variability in surveillance capacity throughout Southeast Asia, and by the fact that statistics may be skewed by underreporting as many who are infected yet experience less intense symptoms may not seek medical assistance, and therefore go unreported.

89. Shortridge et al. 2003.

90. Taubenberger and Morens 2006, p. 21.

91. Robert Weilaard, "EU considers Europe-wide bird flu plan," Associated Press, February 20, 2006.

92. Ibid.

93. Alexander Higgins, "WHO: Bird flu bigger challenge than AIDS," Associated Press, March 6, 2006.

94. Associated Press, "UN pushing bird flu prevention," February 17, 2006.

95. Ibid.

96. Weilaard, "EU Considers Europe-wide bird flu plan."

97. Anthony Mitchell, "WHO: Africa needs to prepare for bird flu," Associated Press, March 9, 2006.

98. Dulue Mbacha, "Wall of distrust in Nigeria bird flu fight," Associated Press, March 1, 2006.

99. Mike Stobbe, "Leavitt: Second bird flu vaccine in works," Associated Press, March 6, 2006.

100. Associated Press, "More Tamiflu ordered for federal stockpile," March 2, 2006.

101. Bruce Finley, "Facing the virus," *Denver Post*, March 6, 2006.

102. Ibid.

103. Thompson and Tebbens 2007.

104. Higgins, "WHO: Bird flu bigger challenge than AIDS."

105. Ibid.

106. The US Congress has historically invoked the Commerce Clause in order to claim jurisdiction over the regulation of environmental issues.

107. "Social capital' refers to "connections among individuals –social networks and the norms of reciprocity and trustworthiness that arise from them" (Putnam 2000, p. 19).

Chapter 4

1. This chapter is based in part on Price-Smith and Daly 2004.

2. UNAIDS, 2006 Report on the Global AIDS Epidemic. www.unaids.org.

3. UNIAIDS, 2006, Epidemic Update, 2006. http://data.unaids.org.

4. UNAIDS, 2006 Report on the Global AIDS Epidemic. http://data.unaids.org.

5. Maclean 2002.

6. UNAIDS, 2006 Report on the Global AIDS Epidemic.

7. Process tracing is widely employed within the emergent school of "environmental security," which seeks to analyze the paths to outcomes as being equally relevant as the outcomes themselves. See Homer-Dixon 1999. The utility of case studies is discussed in Fearon and Laitin 2000. See also Kaufman 2006.

8. Jervis 1997, p. 6.

9. Sprout and Sprout 1968, p.55.

10. Jervis 1997, p. 29.

11. McNeill 1977, p. 61.

12. See Elbe 2002; Ostergard 2002; Price-Smith 2002.

13. In Zimbabwe about 75% of HIV-positive individuals are co-infected with tuberculosis.

14. See Ostergard 2002; Elbe 2002.

15. Price-Smith 2002b.

16. Bloom and Mahal 1997; Bloom and Canning 2000; Price-Smith 2002a.

17. The argument that HIV presents a substantive threat contradicts the emerging constructionist literature which holds that health security arguments are merely artifices fashioned to generate the political will sufficient to tackle problematic global public health issues. See Elbe 2006a.

18. HIV seroprevalence has declined to 1.4% in Thailand and to 6.7% in Uganda. See UNAIDS 2006a.

19. SC can be empirically measured according to the index of measures developed on pp. 25–29 of Price-Smith 2002a.

20. Price-Smith 2002a, chapters 1 and 2.

21. Ostergard 2002, p. 334.

22. UNAIDS, Annex 2:HIV/AIDS Estimates and Data, 2005 and 2003, pp. 505–510. http://data.unaids.org.

23. Claire Bisseker, "AIDS epidemic runs wild," *Financial Mail* (Zimbabwe), July 5, 2002.

24. www.worldbank.org.

25. www.unicef.org.

26. Fourie and Schonteich 2001.

27. UNAIDS, *Annex 2*, 2006.

28. National Intelligence Council 2000, p. 61.

29. Schonteich 1999, p. 57.

30. Bollinger et al. 1999, pp. 3–4.

31. Murray and Lopez 1996.

32. John Robertson, "Zimbabwe's economy shipwrecked." *Times* (London), March 6, 2002.

33. Malcolm F. McPherson, Macroeconomic Models of the Impact of HIV/AIDS, http://ksg.harvard.edu.

34. Ibid.

35. Haacker 2002, p. 35.

36. Bonnel 2000.

37. World data tables, www.worldbank.org.

38. Ibid.

39. FAO, FAO/WFP Crop and Food Supply Assessment Mission to Zimbabwe, June 1, 2001. www.fao.org.

40. Source of data: http://www.businessmap.co.

41. McPherson, Macroeconomic Models.

42. Ibid.

43. Ibid.

44. Data compiled by the author from 2001 and 1995 Interpol International Crime Statistics on Zimbabwe. More recent figures remain unavailable.

45. Makumbe 1997.

46. Zimbabwe: Recent Economic Developments, Selected Issues and Statistical Appendix. IMF Country Report No. 01/13 (January 2001). http://www.imf .org.

47. In the early years of the epidemic, many successful African males contracted HIV as a result of the social norm that wealthy males were expected to have many female sexual partners. In latter years the epidemic's demographic distribution has seen the infection of Zimbabwean society en masse.

48. Daly 2001.

49. Deborah L. Toler, A different approach needed to fight global AIDS epidemic. Progressive Media Project, January 27, 2000. http://www.progressive. org.

50. See Price-Smith 1999, 2002a.

51. See McNeill 1977; Dols 1977.

52. On the role of scarcity in triggering state-sponsored violence, see Kahl 1998.

53. Raymond Copson, Zimbabwe Backgrounder, December 27, 2001, Congressional Research Service, US Library of Congress, p. 12.

54. See Ostergard 2002; Price-Smith 2002a.

55. See, e.g., Elbe 2006b.

56. Paris 2001, p. 88.

57. The US Central Intelligence Agency's *World Factbook 2002* on Zimbabwe bluntly states: "Ignoring international condemnation, Mugabe rigged the 2002 presidential election to have himself reelected."

58. See Elbe 2002; Ostergard 2002.

59. Elbe 2002, pp. 155–156.

60. Armando Mabuchi, Zimbabwe—Security Information. Institute for Security Studies (South Africa). http://www.iss.co.za.

61. Heinecken 2001, p. 11.

62. Yeager 1996, p. 2.

63. Mabuchi, Zimbabwe—Security Information.

64. Ibid.

65. Price-Smith and Daly 2004.

66. See Gurr 1970.

67. Conventional Realist theory argues that shifts in the relative power of states often precipitate interstate conflict. See Waltz 1979.

68. Ibid.

69. Further cross-national empirical studies will be required to evaluate the general applicability of these axioms.

Chapter 5

1. "About BSE" (February 24, 2007). www.cdc.gov.

2. Becker 2005b, p. 1.

3. Effective calculation of risk, and the attendant problems generated by uncertainty, are explored in Posner 2004, particularly on pp. 171–175 and 189–196. See also Sunstein 2002b; Perrow 1999, pp. 324–328.

4. Posner 2004, p. 168.

5. Sunstein 2002a, p. 61.

6. Posner 2004, p. 169.

7. Fox and Peterson 2004, p. 48.

8. As quoted in ibid., p. 51.

9. Fisher 1998, pp. 220–221.

10. Ibid., pp. 222–223.

11. Sanjuan and Dawson 2003, p. 155.

12. O'Neill 2005, p. 299.

13. Fisher 1998, pp. 221–222.

14. Ibid., p. 224.

15. Fox and Peterson 2004, p. 52.

16. "French minister: No country is safe," COMTEX Newswire, January 7, 2001.

17. BBC, "MPs attack European self-interest on BSE," March 3 1998. http://news.bbc.co.uk.

18. BBC, "Vaccination key issue at farming talks," December 13, 2001. http://www.bbc.co.uk.

19. Image theory and its impact on perception are explored in Jervis 1970.

20. CNN, "UK seeks truce in beef war," October 28, 1999. http://money.cnn.com.

21. *Time Europe*, "France: The politics of panic," November 20, 2000. www.time.com.

22. See Bulletin of the European Union 3–2002, "Commission v France (BSE)," Case C-1/00, Decisions by the Court of Justice and the Court of First Instance. http://europa.eu.

23. Patrick Messerlin, "Mad Cow" Disease, France and Europe. Brookings Institution, March 1, 2002. http://www.brookings.edu.

24. Setbon et al. 2005, p. 813.

25. Ibid., p. 814.

26. Ibid., p. 814.

27. Ibid., p. 813.

28. Ibid., p. 824.

29. Messerlin, "Mad Cow" Disease, p. 2.

30. O'Neill 2005, p. 300.

31. In the domain of economics a public bad is typically defined as a good that produces socially undesirable outcomes. Although the principle has historically been employed in the context of externalities such as pollution, it is equally applicable to the emergence and proliferation of infectious disease. See, e.g., Copeland and Taylor 1995.

32. Fox and Peterson 2004, p. 51.

33. Messerlin, "Mad Cow" Disease, p. 2.

34. Krapohl 2003.

35. Krapohl 2005, p. 19.

36. Messerlin, "Mad Cow" Disease, p. 2.

37. Krapohl 2004.

38. Reuters, "Saudi bans beef, mutton imports from EU," January 7, 2001.

39. Ahearn 2005, p. 8.

40. Cohen et al. 2001.

41. Leiss 2003.

42. The initial US ban was only partial.

43. Becker 2005b, p. 4.

44. O'Neill 2005, p. 301.

45. See *Ranchers Cattlemen Action Legal Fund USA vs. USDA* (CV-04–51–BLG-RFC).

46. Becker 2005b, p. 5.

47. Becker 2005a, p. 7.

48. Cited in Becker 2005b, p. 5.

49. CDC, *About BSE*, 2007, p. 2.

50. O'Neill 2005, p. 305.

51. Fox and Peterson 2004, p. 54.

52. O'Neill 2005, p. 304.

53. Becker 2005b, p. 3.

54. Ibid., p. 4.

55. USDA, http://www.ers.usda.gov/news/BSECoverage.htm

56. All data taken from Chicago Mercantile Exchange, March 19, 2007.

57. See Schroeder and Valentin 2005.

58. Data cited in Becker 2005a, p. 4.

59. Sandi Doughton, "Mad-cow scrutiny is scaled way back," *Seattle Times*, February 22, 2007.

60. O'Neill 2005, p. 311.

61. Fox and Peterson 2004, pp. 53–54.

62. O'Neill 2005, p. 309.

63. Becker 2005b, p. 4.

64. Marc Ostfield, Food defense: International Cooperation in a Critical Field of Biodefense, US Department of State, November 30, 2006, p. 2.

65. Kim Yon-se, "Seoul offers US beef concessions," *Korea Times*, February 8, 2007. USDA, http://www.ers.usda.gov/news/BSECoverage.htm.

66. Setbon et al. 2005, p. 823.

67. Redlawsk 2002, p. 1021.

68. See Haas 1990, esp. pp. 50–56. See also Adler 1992.

69. Paarlberg 2000, p. 27.

70. See Haas 1990.

71. See Adler 1992.

72. Youde 2005b.

73. O'Neill 2005, p. 313.

74. Levi and Tetlock 1980. For an expansive treatment of the Rational Actor Model, see Morgenthau 1948.

75. Such refinements are indeed being made by Realists such as Randall Schweller, who are revising the assumptions of the paradigm to explain suboptimal decisions. See, in particular, Schweller 2004.

76. Fisher 1998, p. 221.

Chapter 6

1. WHO, Cumulative Number of Probable Reported Cases of SARS, August 7, 2003, at www.who.int.

2. Peiris et al. 2003.

3. Li et al. 2004.

4. Stephen S. Morse, SARS and the Global Risk of Emerging Infectious Diseases, International Relations and Security Network, 2006, http://www.isn.ethz.ch.

5. On the adverse effects of affect (specifically fear) in decision making, see Jervis 2005, pp. 1–32.

6. Prescott 2003, p. 211.

7. Curley and Thomas 2004; Fidler 2004.

8. Huang 2003a, p. 65.

9. WHO, Cumulative Number of Probable Reported Cases of SARS, August 7, 2003, at www.who.int.

10. Huang 2003a, p. 66.

11. Fidler 2004, p. 75.

12. J. Pomfret, "Official says China erred on outbreak; rare apology cites 'poor coordination,'" *Washington Post*, April 5, 2003.

13. J. Pomfret, "Doctor says Health Ministry lied about disease," *Washington Post*, April 10, 2003.

14. J. Pomfret, "Underreporting, secrecy fuel SARS in Beijing, WHO says." *Washington Post*, April 17, 2003.

15. Fidler 2004, p. 98.

16. Thomas Tsang, cited in K. Bradsher and L. Altman, "Isolation, an old medical tool, has SARS fading," *New York Times*, June 21, 2003.

17. Wong 2006.

18. John Pomfret, "China cites 180 More SARS cases, five deaths," *Washington Post*, April 26, 2003.

19. Cited in Huang 2003a.

20. http://www.who.int/csr/don/2003_07_04/en/.

21. *Far Eastern Economic Review*, April 24, 2004.

22. Catherine Porter, "SARS toll on the film industry: $163 million," *Toronto Star*, March 9, 2004.

23. Ibid.

24. "SARS cost Canadian tourism close to $1 billion," Canadian Press, November 9, 2003, www.ctv.ca.

25. Bruce Little, "Was there a recession in Ontario?" *Globe and Mail*, January 27, 2004.

26. Ibid.

27. Ibid.

28. Lee and McKibben 2003.

29. Asian Development Bank, ERD Policy Brief No. 15, May 2003. See also US General Accounting Office, Emerging Infectious Diseases: Asian SARS Outbreak Challenged International and National Responses, Report to the Chairman,

Subcommittee on Asia and the Pacific, Committee on International Relations, House of Representatives, April 2004, p. 57.

30. He provincial Commission of Inquiry into the SARS epidemic was led by Justice Archie Campbell. The above data are taken from the authors interviews with Justice Campbell pending the completion of his investigation.

31. Prescott 2003, p. 218.

32. See Learning from SARS: Renewal of Public Health in Canada, National Advisory Committee on SARS and Public Health, Health Canada, 2003.

33. Hirschman 1991.

34. Personal conversation with Dr. Huang, April 15, 2005.

35. Reuters, April 23, 2003.

36. The constituent members of ASEAN are Brunei, Cambodia, Indonesia, Laos, Malaysia, Myanmar, Philippines, Singapore, Thailand, and Vietnam.

37. Vatikiotis 2003.

38. "ASEAN + 3": the ten member states of ASEAN plus China, Japan, and South Korea.

39. *People's Daily*, April 30, 2003.

40. Vatikiotis 2003.

41. Ibid.

42. Cheow 2003, p. 2.

43. Morse 1993.

44. For example, the pathogen that causes Legionnaires' Disease evolved within air conditioning units in the US, and the Bovine Spongiform Encephalopathy prion evolved as a result of poor animal husbandry practices in the United Kingdom, both G-8 countries of high capacity. Certain pathogens are actually the products of highly advanced medical environments, for example Vancomycin-resistent enteroccoci (VRE) is the product of the US hospital system and its overuse of antibiotics. Methycillin-resistant staphylococcusaureus (MRSA) is similarly an exclusive product of the North American medical environment. See Baba et al. 2002.

45. Preliminary conclusion of the Campbell commission (personal communication with Justice Archie Campbell).

46. Historical examples include Hamburg's efforts to hide its 17,000 cholera victims to keep its harbor open in 1892 and the US news blackout during the 1918 influenza pandemic for fear of its negative impact on US war efforts. See Donald McNeil Jr., "The next generation of diseases are in hiding, somewhere," *New York Times*, December 28, 2003; Barry 2005.

47. David Heynmann, "Foreword," in Fidler 2004, p. xiii.

48. World Health Assembly, *Revision of the International Health Regulations.* WHA56.28, May 28, 2003.

49. Fidler 2004, p. 133.

50. Source of full text of International Health Regulations (2005): www.who.int.

51. See Price-Smith and Daly 2004; Price-Smith 2002b.

52. Stephen S. Morse, "Factors in the emergence of infectious diseases," in Price-Smith 2001.

53. Archie Campbell, The SARS Commission, Final Report, Ontario Ministry of Health), January 9, 2007, www.sarscommission.ca.

54. Price-Smith 2001.

Chapter 7

1. See Price-Smith 2002a, p. 40.

2. See, e.g., Farmer 2003.

3. Price-Smith 2002a, pp. 141–170.

4. Political science typically utilizes a definition of war based on a conflict that exhibited 1,000 or more battle deaths—a rather arbitrary definition, to say the least, yet commonly accepted. See J. Singer and M. Small, Correlates of War Project: International and Civil War Data, 1816–1992, at http://webapp.icpsr.umich.edu.

5. Cooter 2003, p. 283.

6. Morse 1995.

7. Foege 2000, p. 4.

8. Garfield and Neugut 2000, pp. 32, 33.

9. Zinsser 1934, p. 132.

10. Foege 2000, p. 4.

11. Smallman-Raynor and Cliff 2002, pp. 241.

12. Ibid., p. 242.

13. Toole 2000.

14. Ewald 1994, p. 110.

15. See Prinzing 1916.

16. Slack 1992, p. 7.

17. Hays 2003, p. 71.

18. As was noted above, the term "plague" was used in many contexts to denote epidemic disease resulting from various and diverse forms of pathogens, and current epidemiological evidence suggests that the Plague of Athens resulted from typhus.

19. Thucydides 1980, pp. 40–48. Prinzing (1916, p. 11) argues that war refugees inflated the population of Athens to over 400,000 during this period.

20. Zinsser 1934, p. 120.

21. Ibid., pp. 121–122.

22. Hays 2003, p. 70.

23. McNeill 1977, p. 194.

24. Prinzing 1916, p. 23.

25. Ibid., p. 24.

26. Seitz 1847, p. 55.

27. Prinzing 1916, p. 76.

28. Bavaro et al. 2005, p. 49.

29. Prinzing 1916, p. 117.

30. H. Goden, *Erfahrungen und Ansichten zur Lehre vom Typhus*, Archiv fur mediz. Erfahrung, 1814, p. 342. Translated in Prinzing 1916, p. 121.

31. H. Haser, *Lehrbuch der Geschichte der Medizin und der epidemischen Krankheiten*, volume iii, Third edition, Jena, 1882, p. 612. Translated in Prinzing, pp. 123–4.

32. Woodward 1973, pp. 583–594.

33. See Woodward 1973 and Brown et al. 2004.

34. Bavaro et al. 2005, p. 49. See also Scoville 1948.

35. Bavaro et al. 2005, p. 53.

36. Fuller and Smadel 1954.

37. Hopkins 2002, pp. 103, 104.

38. Prinzing 1916, p. 12.

39. Hopkins 2002, p. 167.

40. Ibid., p. 26.

41. Oldstone 1998, p. 5.

42. Ibid., p. 34.

43. Jefferson, as quoted in Tucker 2001, p. 21.

44. Oldstone 1998, p. 34.

45. Fenn 2004, p. 108.

46. Prinzing 1916, pp. 207, 284.

47. Laveran 1875, p. 364.

48. Rolleston 1933.

49. Evans 2005, p. 223.

50. Guttstadt 1973.

51. Smallman-Raynor and Cliff 2002, p. 262.

52. Ibid., p. 263.

53. Zinsser 1934, pp. 274–275.

54. Hirsch 1883, pp. 503–504.

55. Hays 2003, p. 183.

56. Letgers et al. 1970; Burkle 1973. See also Tikhonov 1999, pp. 23–24.

57. Evans 1992, p. 160.

58. McNeill 1977, p. 233.

59. Hirsch 1883, p. 398.

60. Evans 1992 p. 161.

61. Prinzing 1916, p. 186.

62. Smallman-Raynor and Cliff 2000, p. 29.

63. McNeill 1977, p. 255.

64. Oxford et al. 2002.

65. Ewald 1994, 112.

66. Crosby 2003a.

67. Khan and Laaser, p. 246.

68. Ibid., p. 246.

69. Khan and Laaser 2002, p. 245.

70. Malakooti et al. 1998. See also Matson 1957.

71. Prinzing 1916, p. 195.

72. McNeill 1977, p. 251.

73. See Crosby 1986.

74. Baker and Armelagos 1988.

75. Watts 2003, p. 105.

76. Prinzing 1916, pp. 16–17; Hopkins 2002, p. 29.

77. McNeill 1977, p. 194.

78. Smallman-Raynor and Cliff 1991, p. 69.

79. Lemey et al. 2003, p. 6591.

80. Heinecken 2001.

81. Elbe 2002, p. 163.

82. Pharaoh and Schonteich 2003. http://www.issafrica.org.

83. Elbe 2002, p. 169.

84. Ibid., p. 171.

85. All data from Barnes 1870–1888.

86. Grant and Jorgenson 1995, pp. 1–11.

87. Collier 2003.

88. Toole et al. 1993, p. 1193.

89. Ghobarah et al. 2003, p. 200.

90. Garenne et al. 1997, pp. 318–323.

91. Ghobarah et al. 2003, p. 197.

92. Seaman et al. 1996, p. 864.

93. Ibid., p. 864.

94. Ibid., p. 868.

95. Rey et al. 2002.

96. Ndihokubwayo and Raoult 1999, p. 181.

97. Toole and Waldman 1993, p. 601.

98. Ghobarah et al. 2003, p. 192.

99. Smallman-Raynor and Cliff 2002, pp. 262–263.

100. Przeworski et al. 2000, chapter 4.

101. Ewald 1994, p. 115.

Chapter 8

1. See Deudney 2007, p. 6. As Deudney notes, the term 'Realpolitik' was coined in 1853 by the German Ludwig von Rochau, and the term 'Liberal' arose in the wake of the French Revolution. See also de Bertier de Sauvigny 1970.

2. See McNeill 1977; Diamond 1999; Ranger and Slack 1992; Prinzing 1916; Zinsser 1934; Watts 1997.

3. See Pirages 1995; Price-Smith 1999.

4. Pirages 1995.

5. National Intelligence Council 2000, p. 5.

6. Barton Gellman, "AIDS is declared threat to security: White House fears epidemic could destabilize world," *Washington Post*, April 30, 2000.

7. Al Gore, "Text: Vice President Gore's remarks on AIDS to UN Security Council," January 10, 2000. www.aegis.com.

8. Colin Powell, "Text: Powell address at UN Special Session on HIV/AIDS," June 25, 2001. http://usinfo.state.gov.

9. US Department of State, "Text: Under Secretary Dobriansky on US role in global AIDS struggle," June 22, 2001. http://usinfo.state.gov.

10. Elbe 2002.

11. Ostergard 2002.

12. Singer 2002, p. 145.

13. Peterson 2002–03.

14. Brower and Chalk 2003, p. 101.

15. Price-Smith and Daly 2004.

16. Youde 2005; Peterson and Shellman 2006; Ostergard 2007; Price-Smith 2007.

17. This echoes the fate of the environment-and-security agenda which was similarly dismissed in the post-9/11 era.

18. Morgenthau 1993, p. 30.

19. For example, malaria, which is endemic to tropical regions is unlikely to manifest in significant form within sub-artic and northern temperate regions.

20. This argument echoes McNeill 1977, Crosby 1986, and Landes 1999.

21. Machiavelli's treatise *The Prince* is still widely regarded as a seminal work in the tradition of republican thought, and thus of Classical Realism.

22. Despite the fact that IHR originally appear to have emerged from a materialistic, great-power based, and state-centric constellation of interests, this does not preclude the evolution of the IHR into a norm and process-based regime that reflects the increasing influence of epistemic communities. On power and interest (versus norms and epistemic communities), see Strange 1982; Schweller and Priess 1997; Halabi 2004.

23. Rosen 1993, p. 86.

24. See, e.g., Petty 1899; Graunt 1662.

25. Noted in Rosen 1993, p. 94. See also Seckendorff 1976.

26. Hays 2003, pp. 278–279.

27. Curtin 1989, p. 104.

28. Hays 2003, p. 282.

29. Ibid., p. 279.

30. See, e.g., Howell 2000; Mort 2000; Walkowitz 1982.

31. Hays 2003, p. 280.

32. Doubtless this is related to two factors, the development of antibiotics which have lulled populations into the delusion that microbes are readily controlled, and the recent successes of the Galenic school in discrediting their epistemic rivals.

33. Daniel Deudney has also noted this tendency of modern political scientists to ignore the common Republican tradition which forms the basis for the plethora of modern theories of international relations. See, in particular, Deudney 2007.

34. Ullman 1983, p. 129.

35. Ibid., p. 123.

36. Parson 2003.

37. See Buzan 1991.

38. Ibid., pp. 19–20.

39. Kolodziej 1992, pp. 421–483.

40. Holsti 1996.

41. Ibid., pp. 15–16.

42. Endogenous threats include climate-induced destruction of agriculture, water scarcity, ethnic or religious conflict, and disease.

43. See Homer-Dixon 1999; Hauge and Ellingsen 1998; Deudney and Matthew 1999; Butts 1996; Gleick 1993; Lowi 1993.

44. Here we see an example of how low-tech social ingenuity may in fact provide greater capacity for successful adaptive response than the technical ingenuity (and purely technical responses) of which modern society is so enamored.

45. McLuhan 1969, 1994.

46. See also Peterson and Shellman 2006.

47. Jervis 1976, p. 66.

48. Schweller 2004; Molloy 2003; George 1972.

49. The seminal critique of the unitary-actor hypothesis is Allison 1992. See also Welch 1992; Putnam 1988.

50. Walt 1999.

51. Herbert Simon coined the term 'bounded rationality'. His advances detailing processes of cognition in political decision making are seminal.

52. Jervis 1976, pp. 1–31 in particular.

53. See Tetlock 2000; Ottati et al. 1992.

54. E.g., education, health care, law enforcement, sanitation.

55. In fact, the author proposed such criteria for the securitization of pathogens at the International Studies Association–West meetings in the spring of 2006. There ensued a wonderful debate with the political scientist Sandra MacLean, who argued that such criteria were far too restrictive, and failed to include diseases such as measles.

Conclusion

1. After Alexander Fleming's discovery of penicillin in 1928, human societies began their phase of mastery over the microbial realm. Unfortunately, this era is coming to an end as pathogens have developed powerful capacities for resistance to our antibiotic armamentarium. Viruses, of course, are not affected by antibiotics.

2. The exception to the rule here is Stefan Elbe's excellent work on the various and sundry abuses of "biopower" and "biopolitics" by the state. See Elbe 2006a.

3. This discussion emanates from the debate with my esteemed colleague Sandra MacLean at the ISA-West convention on September 28, 2006. Diseases that destroy the very young and elderly are certainly candidates for threats to human security, but that is beyond the purview of this particular exercise.

4. McNeill 1977, p. 2.

5. This finding also challenges orthodox Realist assumptions, as that body of theory holds that shifts in relative power are associated with inter-state warfare.

6. Increasing prosperity *may* then be transformed into gains in population health. However, this is very much dependent on the equitable distribution of such economic gains in a given polity. As Simon Szreter notes, history provides evidence that macro-level increases in prosperity do *not* always result in increasing population health. See Szreter 2001.

7. Based on author's interview with Stephen S. Morse in Washington DC, July 11, 2007.

8. The rapid revision of the IHR in the wake of SARS suggests a possible exception, however such revisions still took approximately two years after SARS to accomplish.

9. On bio-social negative feedback loops, see Jervis 1997, pp. 134–135.

10. Robert Jervis has explored the fallacy of "games against nature" as if nature was fixed in *System Effects* (1997, p. 48). See also Thompson 1994 and Darwin 2003.

11. The term 'public bad' is derived from Fearon and Laitin 2004.

12. On such policies of denial, see Youde 2007.

13. Price-Smith 2002a.

14. A "society of states" cooperating in this regard is the optimal way to generate global public goods such as surveillance and containment. See Bull 1977; Smith et al. 2003; Conceicao et al. 2003.

15. See http://www.who.int/csr/ihr/en/.

16. Based on author's conversation with Mark Blythe of Johns Hopkins University on January 15, 2007.

17. Author's conversation with Stephen S. Morse of Columbia University, July 11, 2007.

Bibliography

Abu-Lughod, J. 1971. *Cairo: 1001 Years of the City Victorious*. Princeton University Press.

Ackernecht, E. 1948. Anticontagionism between 1821 and 1867. *Bulletin of the History of Medicine* 22, no. 5: 562–593.

Adler, E. 1992. The emergence of co-operation: National epistemic communities and the international evolution of the idea of nuclear arms control. *International Organization* 46, no. 1: 101–145.

Aginam, O. 2005. *Global Health Governance: International Law and Public Health in a Divided World*. University of Toronto Press.

Ahearn, R. 2005. US-European Union Trade Relations: Issues and Policy Challenges, Congressional Research Service Issue Brief IB 10087.

Allen, P. 1979. The "Justiniac" plague. *Byzantion* 49: 5–20.

Allison, G. 1992. *Essence of Decision*. Harper Collins.

Anderson, P. 1972. More is different: Broken symmetry and the nature of the hierarchical structure of science. *Science* 177: 393–396.

Anker, M., and D. Schaaf. 2000. WHO Report on Global Surveillance of Epidemic-Prone Infectious Diseases. Report WHO/CDS/CSR/ISR/2000.1, World Health Organization.

Aristotle. 1984. *Physics*, II v (197a11–13). In *Complete Works of Aristotle*, volume 1, ed. J. Barnes. Princeton University Press.

Aron, J., and J. Patz, eds. 2001. *Ecosystem Change and Public Health: A Global Perspective*. Johns Hopkins University Press.

Ayalon, D. 1946. The plague and its effects upon the Mamluk army. *Journal of the Royal Asiatic Society* 66: 67–73.

Ayres, L. 1919. *The War with Germany: A Statistical Summary*. US Government Printing Office.

Baba, T., et al. 2002. Genome and virulence determinants of high-virulence community-acquired MRSA, *Lancet* 359, no. 9320: 1819–1827.

Bacon, F. 1605. *The Advancement of Learning*.

Bacon, F. 1620. *Novum Organum.*

Bainbridge, W. 1921. Some lessons of the World War in medicine and surgery from the German viewpoint. *Military Surgeon* 49, October: 384–388.

Baker, B., and G. Armelagos. 1988. Origin and antiquity of syphilis: A paleopathological diagnosis and interpretation. *Current Anthropology* 29, no. 5: 703–737.

Baker, T. 1968. Yellowjack: The yellow fever epidemic of 1878 in Memphis, Tennessee. *Bulletin of the History of Medicine* 42: 241–264.

Baldwin, P. 2005. *Contagion and the State in Europe, 1830–1930.* Cambridge University Press.

Barnes, J. 1870–1888. *The Medical and Surgical History of the War of the Rebellion (1861–5)*, volumes 1–3. US Army.

Barry, J. 2005. *The Great Influenza: The Epic Story of the Deadliest Plague in History.* Viking.

Bartlett, M. 1960. The critical community size for measles in the United States. *Journal of the Royal Statistical Society* 123, no. 1: 37–44.

Baumgartner, F., and B. Jones. 2002. *Policy Dynamics.* University of Chicago Press.

Bavaro, M., et al. 2005. History of US military contributions to the study of rickettsial diseases. *Military Medicine* 170, no. 4 (supplement): 49–59.

Becker, G. 2005a. Bovine Spongiform Encephalopathy (Mad Cow Disease): Agricultural Issues for Congress. Issue brief 10127, Congressional Research Service. US Government Printing Office.

Becker, G. 2005b. BSE ("Mad Cow Disease"): A Brief Overview. Report RS22345, Congressional Research Service. US Government Printing Office.

Bessel, R. 1993. *Germany after the First World War.* Clarendon.

Beyerchen, A. 1992–93. Clausewitz, nonlinearity, and the unpredictability of war. *International Security* 17, winter: 59–90.

Bhagwati, J. 2004. *In Defense of Globalization.* Oxford University Press.

Biraben, J.-N. 1976. *Les Hommes et la Peste en France et dans les pays europeens et mediterraneens*, volume 2. Mouton.

Biraben, J.-N., and J. Le Goff. 1969. Le peste dans le haute moyen age. *Annales* 24, no. 6: 1484–1510.

Bloom, D., and D. Canning. 2000. The health and wealth of nations. *Science* 287, February 18: 1207–1209.

Bloom, D., and A. Mahal. 1997. Does the AIDS epidemic threaten economic growth? *Journal of Econometrics* 77, no. 1: 105–124.

Bloom, K. 1993. *The Mississippi Valley's Great Yellow Fever Epidemic of 1878.* Louisiana State University Press.

Blyth, M. 2002. *Great Transformations: Economic Ideas and Institutional Change in the Twentieth Century.* Cambridge University Press.

Bollinger, L., and J. Stover. 1999. *The Economic Impact of AIDS*. Futures Group International.

Bollinger, L., et al. 1999. *The Economic Impact of AIDS in Zimbabwe*. POLICY Project, USAID.

Bonnel, R. 2000. Economic Analysis of HIV/AIDS. ADF2000 background paper, World Bank.

Braudel, F. 1980. *On History*. University of Chicago Press.

Braudel, F. 1993. *A History of Civilizations*. Penguin.

Breunig, C., and C. Koski. 2006. Punctuated equilibrium and budgets in the American states. *Policy Studies Journal* 34, no. 4: 363–379.

Brinkley, J. 2002. Zimbabwe and the Politics of Torture. Special report 92, United States Institute of Peace. http://www.usip.org.

Brower, J., and P. Chalk. 2003. *The Global Threat of New and Reemerging Infectious Diseases: Reconciling US National Security and Public Health Policy*. RAND Corporation.

Brown, A., et al. 2004. Diseases transmitted by arthropod vectors: Typhus. In *Military Preventive Medicine*, ed. P. Kelley. Office of the Surgeon General, Department of the Army.

Brown, C. 1987. The influenza pandemic of 1918 in Indonesia. In *Death and Disease in Southeast Asia*, ed. N. Owen. Oxford University Press.

Brown, C. 1995. *Serpents in the Sand: Essays on the Nonlinear Nature of Politics and Human Destiny*. University of Michigan Press.

Brunetti, M. 1909. Venezia durante la Peste del 1348. *Ateneo Veneto* 32: 295–296.

Bull, H. 1977. *The Anarchical Society: A Study of Order in World Politics*. Macmillan.

Burkle, F., Jr. 1973. Plague as Seen in South Vietnamese children. *Clinical Pediatrics* 12, no. 5: 291–298.

Butts, K. 1996. National security, the environment and the DOD. *Environmental Change and Security Project Report* (Woodrow Wilson Center) 2: 22–27.

Buzan, B. 1991. *People, States, and Fear: An Agenda for International Security Studies in the Post Cold War Era*. Lynne Rienner.

Buzan, B., and R. Little. 2000. *International Systems in World History*. Oxford University Press.

Byerly, C. 2005. *Fever of War: The Influenza Epidemic in the US Army during World War I*. New York University Press.

Calcott, M. 1984. The challenge of cholera: The last epidemic at Newcastle upon Tyne. *Northern History* 20: 75.

Campbell, A. 1931. *The Black Death and Men of Learning*. Columbia University Press.

Carnegie Endowment for International Peace. 1924. *Preliminary History of the Armistice*. Oxford University Press.

Chandavarkar, R. 1992. Plague panic and epidemic politics in India, 1896–1914. In *Epidemics and Ideas*, ed. T. Ranger and P. Slack. Cambridge University Press.

Cheow, E.. 2003. SARS' Three Lessons for ASEAN and ASEAN +3. PACNET #17B, Center for Strategic and International Studies. www.csis.org.

Chickering, R. 2004. *Imperial Germany and the Great War, 1914–1918*, second ed. Cambridge University Press.

Church, J. 1921. French casualty statistics. *Military Surgeon* 48, February: 384–387.

Cipolla, Carlo. 1977. *Faith, Reason and the Plague in Seventeenth Century Tuscany*. Cornell University Press.

Coffey, B., et al. 2005. The Economic Impact of BSE on the US Beef Industry: Product Value Losses, Regulatory Costs, and Consumer Reactions. Extension Bulletin MF-2678, Kansas State University Agricultural Experiment Station and Cooperative Extension Service.

Coffman, E. 1987. *War to End All Wars*. University of Wisconsin Press.

Cohen, J., et al. 2001. Evaluation of the Potential for Bovine Spongiform Encephalopathy in the United States. Harvard Center for Risk Analysis and Center for Computational Epidemiology, Tuskegee University.

Collier, P. 2003. *Breaking the Conflict Trap: Civil War and Development Policy*. World Bank.

Conceicao, P., et al., eds. 2003. *Providing Global Public Goods: Managing Globalization*. Oxford University Press.

Cook, H. 1989. Policing the health of London: The College of Physicians and the early Stuart monarchy. *Social History of Medicine* 27, no. 2: 1–2.

Cooter, R. 2003. Of war and epidemics: Unnatural couplings, problematic conceptions. *Social History of Medicine* 16, no. 2: 283.

Copeland, B., and M. Taylor. 1995. Trade and transboundary pollution. *American Economic Review* 85, no. 4: 716–737.

Copson, R. 2001. Zimbabwe Backgrounder. Congressional Research Service, Library of Congress.

Cottam, M. 1994. *Images and Intervention: US Policies in Latin America*. University of Pittsburgh Press.

Cottam, M., and R. Cottam. 2001. *Nationalism and Politics: The Political Behavior of Nation States*. Lynne Rienner.

Crosby, A., 1986. *Ecological Imperialism: The Biological Expansion of Europe, 900–1900*. Cambridge University Press.

Crosby, A. 2003a. *America's Forgotten Pandemic: The Influenza of 1918*, second edition. Cambridge University Press.

Crosby, A. 2003b. *The Columbian Exchange: Biological and Cultural Consequences of 1492*, thirtieth anniversary edition. Praeger.

Curley, M., and N. Thomas. 2004. Human security and public health in Southeast Asia: The SARS outbreak. *Australian Journal of International Affairs 58*, no. 1: 17–32.

Curtin, P. 1989. *Death by Migration: Europe's Encounter with the Tropical World in the Nineteenth Century*. Cambridge University Press.

Daly, J. 2001. AIDS in Swaziland: The battle from within. *African Studies Review 44*, no. 1: 21–35.

Darwin, C. 2003. *The Origin of Species*. Signet.

Davis, R., and A. Kimball. 2001. The economics of emerging infections in the Asia-Pacific region: What do we know and what do we need to know? In *Plagues and Politics*, ed. A. Price-Smith. Palgrave/Macmillan.

de Bertier de Sauvigny, G. 1970. Liberalism, nationalism, and socialism: The birth of three words. *Review of Politics 32*, no. 2: 147–166.

Delaporte, F. 1986. *Disease and Civilization: The Cholera in Paris, 1832*. MIT Press.

Denevan, W., ed. 1976. *The Native Population of the Americas in 1492*. University of Wisconsin Press.

Deudney, D. 2006. *Bounding Power: Republican Security Theory from the Polis to the Global Village*. Princeton University Press.

Deudney, D., and R. Matthew. 1999. *Contested Grounds: Security and Conflict in the New Environmental Politics*. State University of New York Press.

Diamond, J. 1999. *Guns, Germs, and Steel: The Fates of Human Societies*. Norton.

Diehl, P., and G. Goertz. 2000. *War and Peace in International Rivalry*. University of Michigan Press.

Dobyns, H. 1966. Estimating aboriginal American population. *Current Anthropology 7*: 395–416.

Dols, M. 1977. *The Black Death in the Middle East*. Princeton University Press.

Dowdle, W. 1998. The principles of disease elimination and eradication. *Bulletin of the World Health Organization 48*: 23–27.

Durey, M. 1979. *Return of the Plague: British Society and the Cholera, 1831–2*. Humanities Press.

Durkheim, E. 1938. *The Rules of Sociological Method*. Free Press.

Dutton, D. 1988. *Worse Than the Disease: Pitfalls of Medical Progress*. Cambridge University Press.

Dyer, Christopher. 2002. *Making a Living in the Middle Ages*. Yale University Press.

Easton, D. 1965. *A Systems Analysis of Political Life*. Wiley.

Elbe, S. 2002. HIV/AIDS and the changing landscape of war in Africa. *International Security* 27, no. 2: 159–177.

Elbe, S. 2006a. Should HIV/AIDS be securitized? The ethical dilemmas of linking HIV/AIDS and security. *International Studies Quarterly* 50, no. 1: 119–144.

Elbe, S. 2006b. HIV/AIDS: A human security challenge for the 21st century. *Whitehead Journal of Diplomacy and International Relations*, winter/spring: 1–13.

El-Najjar, M. 1979. Human treponematosis and tuberculosis: Evidence from the New World. *American Journal of Physical Anthropology* 51: 599–618.

Engelbert, P. 2000. *State Legitimacy and Development in Africa*. Lynne Rienner.

Epstein, P. 2000. Is global warming harmful to health? *Scientific American*, August: 36–43.

Epstein, P. 2001. Climate change and emerging infectious diseases. *Microbes and Infection* 3: 747–754.

Evagrius Scholasticus. 1846. *Ecclesiastical History*. H. G. Bohn.

Evans, C. 1998. Historical background. In *Tuberculosis*, second edition, ed. P. Davies. Chapman and Hall Medical.

Evans, R. 1992. Epidemics and revolutions: Cholera in nineteenth century Europe. In *Epidemics and Ideas*, ed. T. Ranger and P. Slack. Cambridge University Press.

Evans, R. 2005. *Death in Hamburg: Society and Politics in the Cholera Years*. Penguin.

Ewald, P. 1994. *Evolution of Infectious Disease*. Oxford University Press.

Farmer, P. 2003. *Pathologies of Power: Health, Human Rights and the New War on the Poor*. University of California Press.

Farwell, B. 1999. *Over There: The United States in the Great War, 1917–1918*. Norton.

Fearon, J., and D. Laitin. 2000. Violence and the social construction of ethnic identity. *International Organization* 54, no. 4: 845–877.

Fearon, J., and D. Laitin. 2004. Neotrusteeship and the problem of weak states. *International Security* 28, no. 4: 5–43.

Fenn, E. 2000. Biological warfare in eighteenth century North America: Beyond Jeffrey Amherst. *Journal of American History* 86, no. 4: 1552–1580.

Fenn, E. 2004. *Pox Americana: The Great Smallpox Epidemic of 1775–81*. Sutton.

Fenner, F. 1988. *The History of Smallpox and Its Spread around the World*. WHO.

Ferguson, N. 2000. *The Pity of War: Explaining World War I*. Basic Books.

Fergusson, W. 1832. *Letters upon the Cholera Morbus.* Highley.

Fidler, D. 1999. *International Law and Infectious Diseases.* Oxford University Press.

Fidler, D. 2004. *SARS, Governance and the Globalization of Disease.* Palgrave/Macmillan.

Findlay, R., and M. Lundahl. 2006. Demographic shocks and the factor proportions model: From the plague of Justinian to the Black Death. In *Eli Heckscher, International Trade, and Economic History*, ed. M. Lundahl et al. MIT Press.

Fisher, J. 1998. "Cattle Plagues Past and Present: The Mystery of Mad Cow Disease." *Journal of Contemporary History* 33, no. 2: 215–229.

Flinn, M. 1979. Plague in Europe and the Mediterranean countries. *Journal of European Economic History* 8, no. 1: 139–144.

Foege, W. 2000. Arms and public health: A global perspective. In *War and Public Health*, ed. B. Levy and V. Sidel. American Public Health Association.

Formicola, V., Q. Milanesi, and C. Scarsini. 1987. Evidence of spinal tuberculosis at the beginning of the fourth millennium BC from Arena Candide cave (Liguria, Italy). *American Journal of Physical Anthropology* 72: 1–7.

Foster, H. 1976. Assessing the magnitude of disaster. *Professional Geographer* 28: 241–247.

Fourie, P., and M. Schonteich. 2001. Africa's new security threat: HIV/AIDS and human security in southern Africa. *African Security Review* 10, no. 4: 29–57.

Fox, J., and H. Peterson. 2004. Risks and implications of bovine spongiform encephalopathy for the United States: Insights from other countries. *Food Policy* 29: 45–60.

Frost, W. 1918. Statistics of influenza morbidity. *Public Health Records* 33, December 27: 2305–2321.

Fuller, H., and J. Smadel. 1954. Rickettsial diseases and the Korean conflict. In *Recent Advances in Medicine and Surgery Based on Professional Experiences in Japan and Korea* 2. US Army Medical Service Graduate School, Walter Reed Army Medical Center.

Gaddis, J. 1997. History, theory, and common ground. *International Security* 22, no. 1: 75–85.

Galen. 1821–1833. *Medicorum Graecorum Opera Quae Exstant*, ed. C. Kühn. Knobloch.

Galen. 1969. *On the Parts of Medicine.* Akademie-Verlag.

Garenne, M., et al. 1997. Effects of the civil war in central Mozambique and evaluation of the intervention of the International Committee of the Red Cross. *Journal of Tropical Pediatrics* 43, no. 6: 318–323.

Garfield, R., and A. Neugut. 2000. The human consequences of war. In *War and Public Health*, ed. B. Levy and V. Sidel. American Public Health Association.

Garrett, L. 1996. The return of infectious disease. *Foreign Affairs* 75, no. 1: 66–79.

Garrison, F. 1920, The German medical history of the war. *Military Surgeon* 46, April: 437.

George, A. 1972. The case for multiple advocacy in making foreign policy. *American Political Science Review* 66, no. 3: 751–785.

George, A. 1979. Case studies and theory development: The method of structured, focused comparison. In *Diplomacy*, ed. P. Lauren. Free Press.

Ghendon, Y. 1994. Introduction to pandemic influenza through history. *European Journal of Epidemiology* 10, no. 4: 451–453.

Ghobarah, H., et al. 2003. Civil wars kill and maim people—long after the shooting stops. *American Political Science Review* 97, no. 2: 192.

Gilpin, R. 1981. *War and Change in World Politics*. Cambridge University Press.

Glacken, C. 1967. *Traces on the Rhodian Shore: Nature and Culture in Western Thought from Ancient Times to the End of the Eighteenth Century*. University of California Press.

Gleick, P. 1993. Water and conflict: Fresh water resources and international security. *International Security* 18, no. 1: 79–112.

Glyn, I., and J. Glyn. 2004. *The Life and Death of Smallpox*. Cambridge University Press.

Gomme, A. 1967. *Population of Athens in the Fifth and Fourth Centuries B.C.* Argonaut.

Gomme, A. 1981. *An Historical Commentary on Thucydides 5*, ed. A. Andrewes and K. Dover. Oxford University Press.

Gordon, D. 2000. The Global Infectious Disease Threat and Its Implications for the United States. Report NIE 99-17D, Central Intelligence Agency.

Gould, S. 2002. *The Structure of Evolutionary Theory*. Belknap.

Grau, L., and W. Jorgenson. 1995. Medical support in a counter-guerrilla war: Epidemiologic lessons learned in the Soviet-Afghan War. *US Army Medical Department Journal*, May-June: 41–49.

Graunt, J. 1662. *Natural and Political Observations Mentioned in a Following Index, and Made upon the Bills of Mortality*. Roycroft.

Gruzinski, S. 1993. *The Conquest of Mexico: The Incorporation of Indian Societies into the Western World, 16th–18th Centuries*. Polity.

Gurr, T. 1970. *Why Men Rebel*. Princeton University Press.

Guttstadt, A. 1973. Die Pocken-Epidemie in Preussen, insbesondere in Berlin 1870/72, nebst Beitragen zur Beurtheilung der Impffrage. *Zeitschrift des königlich Preussischen Statistischen Bureaus* 13: 116–158.

Haacker, M. 2002. The Economic Consequences of HIV/AIDS in Southern Africa. Working paper WP/02/38, International Monetary Fund.

Haas, E. 1964. *Beyond the Nation-State: Functionalism and International Organization*. Stanford University Press.

Haas, P. 1990. *Saving the Mediterranean: The Politics of International Environmental Cooperation*. Columbia University Press.

Halabi, Y. 2004. The expansion of global governance into the Third World: Altruism, realism or constructivism? *International Studies Review* 6, no. 1: 21–48.

Haser, H. *Lehrbuch der Geschichte der Medizin und der epidemischen Krankheiten*, vol iii, Third edition, Jena, 1882

Hatcher, J., 1977. *Plague, Population and the English Economy, 1348–1530*. Macmillan.

Hauge, W., and T. Ellingsen. 1998. Beyond environmental scarcity: Causal pathways to conflict. *Journal of Peace Research* 35, no. 3: 299–317.

Hays, J. 2003. *The Burdens of Disease: Epidemics and Human Response in Western History*. Rutgers University Press.

Heinecken, L. 2001. Living in terror: The looming security threat to southern Africa. *African Security Review* 10, no. 4: 7–17.

Henderson, D. 1996. Smallpox eradication. In *Microbe Hunters Past and Present*, ed. H. Kaprowski and M. Oldstone. Bloomington.

Hermann, D. 1997. *The Arming of Europe and the Making of the First World War*. Princeton University Press.

Herrmann, R., et al. 1997. Images in international relations: An experimental test of cognitive schemata. *International Studies Quarterly* 41, no. 3: 403–433.

Hildreth, M. 1991. The influenza epidemic of 1918–1919 in France: Contemporary concepts of aetiology, therapy and prevention. *Social History of Medicine* 4. August: 277–294.

Hippocrates. 1994. *Epidemics I and III*. Loeb Classical Library.

Hirsch, A. 1883. *Handbook of Geographical and Historical Pathology*, volume 1: *Acute Infective Diseases*. New Sydenham Society.

Hobbes, T. 1985. *Leviathan*. Penguin.

Hoffman, S. 1961. International systems and international law. In *The International System*, ed. K. Knorr and S. Verba. Princeton University Press.

Holsti, K. 1996. *The State, War, and the State of War*. Cambridge University Press.

Homer-Dixon, T. 1999. *Environment, Scarcity, and Violence*. Princeton University Press.

Homer-Dixon, T. 2000. *The Ingenuity Gap*. Knopf.

Hopkins, D. 1983. *Princes and Peasants: Smallpox in History*. University of Chicago Press.

Hopkins, D. 2002. *The Greatest Killer: Smallpox in History*. University of Chicago Press.

Howell, P. 2000. A private Contagious Diseases Act: Prostitution and public space in Victorian Cambridge. *Journal of Historical Geography* 26, no. 3: 376–402.

Huang, Y. 2003a. The politics of China's SARS Crisis. *Harvard Asia Quarterly* 7, no. 4: 9–16.

Huang, Y. 2003b. Mortal Peril: Public Health in China and Its Security Implications. Health and Security Series Special Report No. 7, Chemical and Biological Arms Control Institute.

Ibn Khaldun, A. 1958. *The Muqaddimah*, volume 1. Pantheon.

Irwin, R. 1986. *The Middle East in the Middle Ages: The Early Mamluk Sultanate 1250–1382*. Southern Illinois University Press.

Jelavich, B. 1983. *History of the Balkans: Eighteenth and Nineteenth Centuries*. Cambridge University Press.

Jervis, R. 1970. *The Logic of Images in International Relations*. Princeton University Press.

Jervis, R. 1976. *Perception and Misperception in International Politics*. Princeton University Press.

Jervis, R. 1997. *System Effects: Complexity in Political and Social Life*. Princeton University Press.

Jervis, R. 2005. *American Foreign Policy in a New Era*. Routledge.

Johnson, N., and J. Mueller. 2002. Updating the accounts: Global mortality of the 1918–1920 "Spanish" influenza pandemic. *Bulletin of the History of Medicine* 76, no. 1: 105–115.

Kahl, C. 1998. Population growth, environmental degradation, and state-sponsored violence: The case of Kenya, 1991–93. *International Security* 23, no. 2: 80–119.

Kahl, C. 2006. *States, Scarcity and Strife in the Developing World*. Princeton University Press.

Kamen, H. 1980. *Spain in the Later 17th Century: 1665–1700*. Longman.

Katzenstein, P. 1978. Conclusion. In *Between Power and Plenty,* ed. P. Katzenstein. University of Wisconsin Press.

Kaufman, S. 2006. Symbolic politics or rational choice. *International Security* 30, no. 4: 45–86.

Kaye, D., and C. Pringle. 2003. Avian influenza viruses and their implications for human health. *Clinical Infectious Diseases* 40: 108–112.

Keegan, J. 2000. *The First World War*. Vintage.

Keene, J. 2001. *Doughboys, the Great War, and the Remaking of America*. Johns Hopkins University Press.

Kelly, D. 1990. *The Human Measure: Social Thought in the Western Legal Tradition*. Harvard University Press.

Kelly, J. 2005. *The Great Mortality.* Harper.

Khan, I., and U. Laaser. 2002. Burden of tuberculosis in Afghanistan: Update on a war-stricken country. *Croatian Medical Journal* 43, no. 2: 245–247.

Kiel, L., and E. Elliot, eds. 1966. *Chaos Theory in the Social Sciences.* University of Michigan Press.

Kolodziej, E. 1992. Renaissance in security studies? Caveat lector! *International Studies Quarterly* 36: 421–483.

Krapohl, S. 2003. Risk regulation in the EU between interests and expertise: The case of BSE. *Journal of European Public Policy* 10, no. 2: 189–207.

Krapohl, S. 2004. Credible commitment in non-independent regulatory agencies. *European Law Journal* 10, no. 5: 518–538.

Krapohl, S. 2005. Thalidomide, BSE and the Single Market. Working paper LAW 2005/03, Department of Law, European University Institute.

Krasner, S. 1978. *Defending the National Interest.* Princeton University Press.

Krasner, S. 1984. Approaches to the state: Alternative conceptions and historical dynamics. *Comparative Politics* 16, no. 2: 223–246.

Krugman, P., and A. Venables. 1995. Globalization and the inequality of nations. *Quarterly Journal of Economics* 110, no. 4: 857–880.

Kuhn, T. 1962. *The Structure of Scientific Revolutions.* University of Chicago Press.

Kwaramba, P. 1997. The Socio-Economic Impact of HIV/AIDS on Communal Agricultural Systems in Zimbabwe. Working paper 19, Zimbabwe Farmers Union, Friedrich Ebert Stiftung Economic Advisory Project, Harare.

Landes, D. 1999. *The Wealth and Poverty of Nations.* Norton.

Laughlin, R. 2005. *A Different Universe: Reinventing Physics from the Bottom Down.* Basic Books.

Laveran, A. 1875. *Traite des Maladies et Epidemies des Armees.* Masson.

Lee, J.-W., and W. McKibben. 2003. Globalization and Disease: The Case of SARS. Working paper 2003/16, Research School of Pacific and Asian Studies, Australian National University and Brookings Institution.

Lederberg, J. 1997. Infectious disease as an evolutionary paradigm. *Emerging Infectious Diseases* 3, no. 4: 1–15.

Leiss, W. 2003. BSE risk in Canada: Finally, the penny drops. *Risk Issue Chronicles* 5: 35–39.

Lemey, P., et al. 2003. Tracing the origin and history of the HIV-2 epidemic. *Proceedings of the National Academy of Sciences* 100: 6591.

Letgers, L., A. Cottingham, and D. Hunter. 1970. Clinical and epidemiological notes on a defined outbreak of plague in Vietnam. *American Journal of Tropical Medicine and Hygiene* 19, no. 4: 639–652.

Levi, A., and P. Tetlock. 1980. A cognitive analysis of Japan's 1941 decisions for war. *Journal of Conflict Resolution* 24, no. 2: 195–211.

Li, K., et al. 2004. Genesis of a highly pathogenic and potentially pandemic H5N1 influenza virus in eastern Asia. *Nature* 430, July 8: 209–213.

Littman, R., and M. Littman. 1973. Galen and the Antonine plague. *American Journal of Philology* 94: 244.

Livesey, A. 1989. *Great Battles of World War I.* Macmillan.

Lockhart, J. 1992. *The Nahuas after the Conquest: A Social and Cultural History of the Indians of Central Mexico, Sixteenth through Eighteenth Centuries.* Stanford University Press.

Lodge, M., and C. Taber. 2005. The automaticity of affect for political leaders, groups, and issues: An experimental test of the Hot Cognition Hypothesis. *Political Psychology* 26, no. 3: 455–482.

Longrigg, J. 1992. Epidemics, ideas, and classical Athenian society. In *Epidemics and Ideas*, ed. T. Ranger and P. Slack. Cambridge University Press.

Lovell, G. 1992. Heavy shadows and black night: Disease and depopulation in colonial Spanish America. *Annals of the Association of American Geographers* 82, no. 3: 435–437.

Lowi, M. 1993. *Water and Power: The Politics of a Scarce Resource in the Jordan River Basin.* Cambridge University Press.

Luckin, B. 1984. States and epidemic threats. *Bulletin of the Social History of Medicine* 34, June: 25–27.

Ludendorff, E. von. 1919. *Ludendorff's Own Story, August 1914–November 1918*, volume 2. Harper.

Maclean, S. 2002. Mugabe at war: The political economy of conflict in Zimbabwe. *Third World Quarterly* 23, no. 3: 513–528.

MacLeod, D. 1992. Microbes and muskets: Smallpox and the participation of the Amerindian allies of New France in the Seven Years War. *Ethnohistory* 31, no. 1: 49–50.

Macmillan, M. 2003. *Paris 1919: Six Months that Changed the World.* Random House.

Makumbe, J. 1997. The Role of Government in Adjusting Economies—The Zimbabwe Civil Service: A Wind of Change. International Development Department (UK).

Malakooti, M., et al. 1998. Resurgence of epidemic malaria in the highlands of western Kenya. *Emerging Infectious Diseases* 4, no. 4: 671–672.

Marcus, G., et al. 2000. *Affective Intelligence and Political Judgment.* University of Chicago Press.

Markel, H. 1993. Cholera, quarantines, and immigration restriction: The view from Johns Hopkins, 1892. *Bulletin of the History of Medicine* 67, no. 4: 691–702.

Matson, A. 1957. The history of malaria in Nandi. *East Africa Medical Journal* 34: 431–441.

McGrew, R. 1965. *Russia and the Cholera: 1823–1832*. University of Wisconsin Press.

McInnes, C. 2006. HIV/AIDS and security. *International Affairs* 82, no. 2: 315–326.

McLuhan, M. 1969. *The Gutenberg Galaxy*. Signet.

McLuhan, M. 1994. *Understanding Media: The Extensions of Man*. MIT Press.

McMichael, A. 2003. *Planetary Overload: Global Environmental Change and the Health of the Human Species*. Cambridge University Press.

McMichael, T. 2001. *Human Frontiers, Environments and Disease*. Cambridge University Press.

McNeill, W. 1977. *Plagues and Peoples*. Anchor.

McNeill, W. 1989. Control and catastrophe in human affairs. *Daedalus*, winter: 1–2.

McNeill, W. 1992. *The Global Condition: Conquerors, Catastrophes, and Community*. Princeton University Press.

Mearshimer, J. 2003. *The Tragedy of Great Power Politics*. Norton.

Mercer, W. 1964. Then and now: History of skeletal tuberculosis. *Journal of the Royal College of Surgeon of Edinburgh* 9: 243–254.

Migdal, J. 1988. *Strong Societies and Weak States: State-Society Relations and State Capabilities in the Third World*. Princeton University Press.

Mills, I. 1986. The 1918–1919 influenza pandemic: The Indian experience. *Indian Economic and Social History Review* 23: 1–40.

National Intelligence Council. 2000. The Global Infectious Disease Threat and Its Implications for the United States.

Moller-Christensen, V. 1969. The history of syphilis and leprosy: An osteo-archological approach. *Abbotempo* 1: 20–25.

Molloy, S. 2003. Realism: A problematic paradigm. *Security Dialogue* 34, no. 1: 71–85.

Monto, A. 2005. The threat of an avian influenza pandemic. *New England Journal of Medicine* 352, no. 4: 323–325.

Morgenthau, H. 1948. *Politics among Nations: The Struggle for Power and Peace*. Knopf.

Morris, J., et al. 2003. Activation of political attitudes: A psychological examination of the Hot Cognition Hypothesis. *Political Psychology* 24, no. 4: 727–745.

Morse, S., ed. 1993. *Emerging Viruses*. Oxford University Press.

Morse, S. 1995. Factors in the emergence of infectious diseases. *Emerging Infectious Diseases* 1, no. 1: 7–15.

Mort, F. 2000. *Dangerous Sexualities: Medicomoral Politics in England since 1830*. Routledge.

Murray, C., and A. Lopez. 1996. *The Global Burden of Disease*. Harvard University Press.

Murrin, J. 1990. Beneficiaries of catastrophe: The English colonies in America. In *The New American History*, ed. E. Foner. Temple University Press.

National Intelligence Council. 2000. National Intelligence Estimate: The Global Infectious Disease Threat and its Implications for the United States. Reprinted in *Environmental Change and Security Project Report*, Report 6, Woodrow Wilson Center, 2000.

Ndihokubwayo, J., and D. Raoult. 1999. Epidemic typhus in Africa. *Medicene Tropical (Mars)* 59, no. 2: 181.

Nohl, J. 2006. *The Black Death: A Chronicle of the Plague*. Westholme.

North, D. 1990. *Institutions, Institutional Change and Economic Performance*. Cambridge University Press.

Noymer, A., and M. Garenne. 2003. Long-term effects of the 1918 "Spanish" influenza epidemic on sex differentials of mortality in the USA. In *The Spanish Influenza Pandemic of 1918–1919*, ed. H. Philips and D. Killingray. Routledge.

Oestrich, G. 1982. *Neostoicism and the Early Modern State*. Cambridge University Press.

Oldstone, M. 1998. *Viruses, Plagues and History*. Oxford University Press.

O'Neill, Kate. 2005. How two cows make a crisis: US-Canada trade relations and Mad Cow Disease. *American Review of Canadian Studies*, summer: 299.

Onuf, N. 1998. *The Republican Legacy in International Thought*. Cambridge University Press.

O'Rourke, K., and J. Williamson. 2001. *Globalization and History: The Evolution of a Nineteenth Century Atlantic Economy*. MIT Press.

Ostergard, R., Jr. 2002. Politics in the Hot Zone: AIDS and national security in Africa. *Third World Quarterly* 23, no. 2: 333–350.

Ottati, V., et al. 1992. The cognitive and affective components of political attitudes. *Political Behavior* 14, no. 4: 423–442.

Oxford, J., et al. 2002. World War I may have allowed the emergence of "Spanish" influenza. *Lancet Infectious Diseases* 2, no. 2: 111–114.

Oxford, J., et al. 2005. A hypothesis: The conjunction of soldiers, gas, pigs, ducks, geese and horses in northern France during the Great War provided the conditions for the emergence of the "Spanish" influenza pandemic of 1918–1919. *Vaccine* 23, no. 7: 940–945.

Paarlberg, E. 2000. The global food fight. *Foreign Affairs* 79, no. 3: 24–38.

Palmer, R. 1993. *English Law in the Age of the Black Death: A Transformation of Governance and Law*. University of North Carolina Press.

Papagrigorakis, M., et al. 2006. DNA examination of ancient dental pulp incriminate typhoid fever as a probable cause of the Plague of Athens. *International Journal of Infectious Diseases* 10, no. 3: 206–214.

Paris, R. 2001. Human security: Paradigm shift or hot air. *International Security* 26, no. 2: 87–102.

Parson, E. 2003. *Protecting the Ozone Layer: Science and Strategy.* Oxford University Press.

Patterson, D. 1983. The influenza epidemic of 1918–1919 on the Gold Coast. *Journal of African History* 24: 485–502.

Peiris, J., et al. 2003. Coronavirus as a possible cause of severe acute respiratory syndrome. *Lancet* 361, no. 9366: 1319–1325.

Perrow, C. 1999. *Normal Accidents: Living with High-Risk Technologies,* second edition. Princeton University Press.

Peterson, S. 2002–03. Epidemic disease and national security. *Security Studies* 12, no. 2: 43–80.

Petty, W. 1899. *The Economic Writings of Sir William Petty, together with Observations Upon the Bills of Mortality more probably by Captain John Graunt,* ed. C. Hull. Cambridge University Press.

Pharaoh, R., and M. Schonteich. 2003. AIDS, Security and Governance in Southern Africa: Exploring the Impact. Paper 65, Institute for Security Studies.

Philipps, D. 1976. *Holistic Thought in Social Science.* Stanford University Press.

Phillips, H., and D. Killingray. 2003. *The Spanish Influenza Pandemic of 1918–19: New Perspectives.* Routledge.

Pirages, D. 1995. Microsecurity: Disease organisms and human well-being. *Washington Quarterly* 18, no. 4: 5–12.

Pirages, D. 1996. Microsecurity: Disease organisms and human well-being. In *Environmental Security Project Report.* Environmental Change and Security Project. Woodrow Wilson Center.

Poku, N. 2002. Poverty, debt and Africa's HIV/AIDS Crisis. *International Affairs* 78, no. 3: 531–546.

Posner, R. 2004. *Catastrophe: Risk and Response.* Oxford University Press.

Powell, J. 1993. *Bring Out Your Dead: The Great Plague of Yellow Fever in Philadelphia in 1783.* University of Pennsylvania Press.

Poznansky, A. 1996. *Tchaikovsky's Last Days.* Oxford University Press.

Prescott, E. 2003. SARS: A warning. *Survival* 45, no. 3: 207–225.

Price-Smith, A. 1999. Ghosts of Kigali: Infectious disease and global stability in the coming century. *International Journal* 54, no. 3: 426–442.

Price-Smith, A., ed. 2001. *Plagues and Politics: Infectious Disease and International Policy.* Palgrave/Macmillan.

Price-Smith, A. 2002a. *The Health of Nations: Infectious Disease, Environmental Change and their Effects on National Security and Development.* MIT Press.

Price-Smith, A. 2002b. *Pretoria's Shadow.* Chemical and Biological Arms Control Institute.

Price-Smith, A., and J. Daly. 2004. *Downward Spiral: HIV/AIDS, State Capacity and Political Conflict in Zimbabwe.* United States Institute of Peace Press.

Price-Smith, A., S. Tauber, and A. Bhat. 2004. Preliminary evidence of an empirical association between state capacity and adaptation to HIV/AIDS. *Seton Hall Journal of Diplomacy and International Affairs* 5, no. 2: 149–160.

Prinzing, F. 1916. *Epidemics Resulting from Wars.* Carnegie Endowment for International Peace/Clarendon.

Procopius. 1914. *History of the Wars,* ed. H. Dewing. Harvard University Press.

Przeworski, A., et al. 2000. *Democracy and Development: Political Institutions and Well-Being in the World, 1950–1990.* Cambridge University Press.

Putnam, R. 1988. Diplomacy and domestic politics: The logic of two level games. *International Organization* 42, no. 3: 427–460.

Putnam, R. 2000. *Bowling Alone: The Collapse and Revival of American Community.* Simon & Schuster.

Ranger, T., and P. Slack, eds. 1992. *Epidemics and Ideas.* Cambridge University Press.

Redlawsk, D. 2002. Hot cognition or cool consideration? Testing the effects of motivated reasoning on political decision-making. *Journal of Politics* 64, no. 4: 1021–1044.

Rey, J., et al. 2002. Sero-epidemiological study of the hepatitis epidemic in Mitrovica in the aftermath of the war in Kosovo (1999). *Bulletin de la Societe de Pathologie Exotique* 95, no. 1: 3–7.

Rheinstein, M., ed. 1954. *Max Weber on Law and Economy and Society.* Harvard University Press.

Rice, G. 1983. Maori mortality in the 1918 influenza pandemic. *New Zealand Population Review* 9: 44–61.

Rice, G., and E. Palmer. 1993. Pandemic influenza in Japan: Mortality patterns and official responses. *Journal of Japanese Studies* 19, no. 2: 394.

Richardson, G. 1991. *Feedback Thought in Social Science and Systems Theory.* University of Pennsylvania Press.

Robin, C. 2004. *Fear: The History of a Political Idea.* Oxford University Press.

Rolleston, J. 1933. The smallpox pandemic of 1870–74. *Proceedings of the Royal Society of Medicine, Section of Epidemiology and State Medicine* 27: 177–192.

Romanelli, E., and M. Tushman. 1994. Organizational transformation as punctuated equilibrium: An empirical test. *Academy of Management Journal* 37, no. 5: 1141–1166.

Rosen, G. 1993. *A History of Public Health*. Johns Hopkins University Press.

Rosen, W. 2007. *Justinian's Flea: Plague, Empire, and the Birth of Europe*. Viking.

Rosenau, J. 1997. *Along the Foreign-Domestic Frontier: Exploring Governance in a Turbulent World*. Cambridge University Press.

Rosenberg, C. 1966. Cholera in nineteenth century Europe. *Comparative Studies in Society and History* 8: 452–463.

Rothenberg, G. 1973. The Austrian sanitary cordon and the control of the bubonic plague: 1710–1871. *Journal of the History of Medicine* 28, no. 1: 16–19.

Rousseau, J.-J. 1968. *The Social Contract*. Penguin.

Rousseau, J.-J. 2005. *The Confessions*. Penguin.

Ruffer, M. 1921. Pathological notes on the royal mummies of a Cairo museum. In *Studies in the Paleontology of Egypt*, ed. R. Moodie. University of Chicago Press.

Russell, J. 1968. That earlier plague. *Demography* 5, no. 1: 174–184.

Safranek, T. 1991. Reassessment of the association between Guillain-Barre Syndrome and receipt of swine influenza vaccine in 1976–77: Results of a two-state study. *American Journal of Epidemiology* 133, no. 9: 940–941.

Sanjuan, A., and P. Dawson. 2003. Price transmission, BSE and structural breaks in the UK meat sector. *European Review of Agricultural Economics* 30, no. 2: 155.

Schafer, J., et al. 1993. Origin of the pandemic 1957 H2 influenza A virus. *Virology* 194, no. 2: 781–788.

Schonteich, M. 1999. Age and AIDS: South Africa's crime time bomb? *Africa Security Review* 18, no. 4: 1–4.

Schroeder. T., and L. Valentin. 2005. The Economic Impact of BSE on the US Beef Industry. Working paper MF-2679, Department of Agricultural Economics, Kansas State University.

Schumpeter, J. 2005. *Capitalism, Socialism and Democracy*. Routledge.

Schweller, R. 2004. Unanswered threats: A neoclassical realist theory of underbalancing. *International Security* 29, no. 2: 159–2001.

Schweller, R., and D. Priess. 1997. A tale of two realisms: Expanding the institutions debate. *Mershon International Studies Review* 41, no. 1: 1–32.

Scoville, A. 1948. Epidemic typhus fever in Japan and Korea. In *Rickettsial Diseases of Man*, ed. M. Soule. American Association for the Advancement of Science.

Seaman, J., et al. 1996. The epidemic of visceral leishmaniasis in western upper Nile, southern Sudan: Course and impact from 1984 to 1994. *International Journal of Epidemiology* 25, no. 4: 862–871.

Seckendorff, V. von. 1976. *Teutscher Fursten Stat* (reprint). Auvermann.

Seidule, J. T. 1997. Morale in the American Expeditionary Forces. PhD dissertation, Ohio State University.

Seitz, F. 1847. *Der Typhus, vorzuglich nach seinem Vorkommen in Bayern geshildert*. Erlangen.

Setbon, M., et al. 2005. Risk perception of the "Mad Cow Disease" in France: Determinants and consequences. *Risk Analysis* 25, no. 4: 813–826.

Shatzmiller, J. 1974. Les Juifs de Provence pendant a Peste Noire. *Revue des Etudes Juifes* 133: 457–480.

Shortridge, K., et al. 2003. The next influenza pandemic: Lessons from Hong Kong. *Journal of Applied Microbiology* 94, no. 1: 70–77.

Sigerist, H. 1962. *Civilization and Disease*. University of Chicago Press.

Silverstein, A. 1981. *Pure Politics and Impure Science: The Swine Flu Affair*. Johns Hopkins University Press.

Simon, H. 1983. *Reason in Human Affairs*. Stanford University Press.

Simon, H. 1997, *Models of Bounded Rationality*, volumes 1–3. MIT Press.

Singer, P. W. 2002. AIDS and International Security. *Survival* 44, no. 1: 145–158.

Skocpol, T. 1985. Bringing the state back in: Strategies of analysis in current research. In *Bringing the State Back In*, ed. P. Evans, et al. Cambridge University Press.

Slack, P. 1985. *The Impact of the Plague in Tudor and Stuart England*. Routledge & Kegan Paul.

Slack, P. 1992. Introduction. In *Epidemics and Ideas*, ed. T. Ranger and P. Slack. Cambridge University Press.

Smallman-Raynor, M., and A. Cliff. 1991. Civil war and the spread of AIDS in central Africa. *Epidemiology and Infection* 107, no. 1: 69–73.

Smallman-Raynor, M., and A. Cliff. 2000. The epidemiological legacy of war: The Philippine-American War and the diffusion of cholera in Batangas and La Laguna, South-West Luzon, 1902–1904. *War in History* 7, no. 1: 29.

Smallman-Raynor, M., and A. Cliff. 2002. The geographical transmission of smallpox in the Franco-Prussian War: Prisoner of war camps and their impact upon epidemic diffusion processes in the civil settlement system of Prussia, 1870–71. *Medical History* 46: 241.

Smith, R., et al., eds. 2003. *Global Public Goods for Health*. Oxford University Press.

Snowdon, F. 1995. *Naples in the Time of Cholera, 1884–1911*. Cambridge University Press.

Speth, J., and R. Repetto. 2006. *Punctuated Equilibrium and the Dynamics of US Environmental Policy.* Yale University Press.

Sprout, H. and M. Sprout. 1968. An Ecological Paradigm for the Study of International Politics. Research memorandum 30, Center for International Studies, Princeton University.

Steinbock, R. 1976. *Paleopathological Diagnosis and Interpretation.* Charles Thomas.

Stiglitz, J. 2006. *Making Globalization Work.* Norton.

Stinchcombe, A. 1968. *Constructing Social Theories.* Harcourt Brace.

Strange, S. 1982. Cave! Hic dragones: A critique of regime analysis. *International Organization* 36, no. 2: 479–496.

Strauss, L. 1953. *Natural Right and History.* University of Chicago Press.

Sunstein, C. 2002a. Probability neglect: Emotions, worst cases, and law. *Yale Law Journal* 112, no. 1: 61–108.

Sunstein, C. 2002b. *Risk and Reason: Safety, Law and the Environment.* Cambridge University Press.

Sydenstricker, E. 1918. Preliminary statistics of the influenza epidemic. *Public Health Records,* December 27: 2305–2321.

Szreter, S. 2001. Economic Growth, Disruption, Deprivation, Disease and Death: On the Importance of the Politics of Public Health for Development. In *Plagues and Politics,* ed. A. Price-Smith. Palgrave/Macmillan.

Tainter, J. 1988. *The Collapse of Complex Societies.* Cambridge University Press.

Taubenberger, J. 1999. Seeking the 1918 Spanish influenza virus. *ASM News* 65, July 7: 473.

Taubenberger, J., and D. Morens. 2006. 1918 influenza: The mother of all pandemics. *Emerging Infectious Diseases* 12, no. 1: 15–22.

Tetlock, P. 2000. Cognitive biases and organizational correctives. *Administrative Science Quarterly* 45, no. 2: 293–326.

Thagard, P., and F. Kroon. 2006. *Hot Thought: Mechanisms and Applications of Emotional Cognition.* MIT Press.

Thompson, J. 1994. *The Coevolutionary Process.* University of Chicago Press.

Thompson, K., and R. Tebbens. 2007. Eradication versus control for poliomyelitis: An economic analysis. *Lancet* 369, no. 9570: 1363–1371.

Thornton, R. 1987. *American Indian Holocaust and Survival.* University of Oklahoma Press.

Thucydides. 1980. *History of the Peloponnesian War.* Penguin.

Tomkins, S. 1992. The failure of expertise: Public health policy in Britain during the 1918–19 influenza epidemic. *Social History of Medicine* 5, December: 435–454.

Toole, M., et al. 1993. Are war and public health compatible? *Lancet* 341, May 8: 1193.

Toole, M. 2000. Displaced persons and war. In *War and Public Health*, ed. B. Levy and V. Sidel. APHA.

Toole, M., and R. Waldman. 1993. Refugees and displaced persons: War, hunger, and public health. *JAMA* 270, no. 5: 600–605.

Tucker, J. 2001. *Scourge: The Once and Future Threat of Smallpox*. Grove.

Ullman, R. 1983. Redefining security. *International Security* 8, no. 1: 129–153.

United Nations Development Program. 1994. *New Dimensions of Human Security*. Oxford University Press.

van Evera, S. 2001. *Causes of War*. Cornell University Press.

Vatikiotis, M. 2003. ASEAN and China—united in adversity. *Far Eastern Economic Review*, May 8: 14–17.

Verity, D., et al. 1999. Behcet's Disease, the Silk Road and HLA-B51: Historical and geographical perspectives. *Tissue Antigens* 54, no. 3: 213–220.

Volkmann, E. 1925. *Der Marxismus und des deutsche Heer im Weltkriege*. Hobbing.

Walkowitz, J. 1982. *Prostitution and Victorian Society: Women, Class, and the State*. Cambridge University Press.

Walt, S. 1996. Rethinking revolution and war: A reply to Goldstone and Dassel. *Security Studies* 6, no. 2: 177.

Walt, S. 1999. Rigor or rigor mortis? Rational choice and security studies. *International Security* 23, no. 4: 5–48.

Waltz, K. 1979. *Theory of International Politics*. McGraw-Hill.

Waltz, K. 1990. Nuclear myths and political realities. *American Political Science Review* 84, no. 3: 731–745.

Watts, S. 1997. *Epidemics and History: Disease, Power and Imperialism*. Yale University Press.

Watts, S. 2003. *Disease and Medicine in World History*. Routledge.

Weber, M. 1964. *The Theory of Social and Economic Organization*, ed. T. Parsons. Free Press.

Welch, D. 1992. The organizational process and bureaucratic politics paradigms: Retrospect and prospect. *International Security* 17, no. 2: 112–146.

Wells, C. 1964. *Bones, Bodies and Disease*. Thames and Hudson.

Wendt, A. 1999. *Social Theory of International Politics*. Cambridge University Press.

Wheelis, M. 1999. Biological warfare before 1914. In *Biological and Toxic Weapons*, ed. E. Geissler and J. Moon. Oxford University Press for SIPRI.

Whewell, W. 1840. *Philosophy of the Inductive Sciences*. John W. Parker.

Whiteside, A. 2002. Poverty and HIV/AIDS in Africa. *Third World Quarterly* 23, no. 2: 313–332.

WHO. 1994. Constitution of the WHO, 1948. In *WHO, Basic Documents*, fortieth edition.

Wilson, E. 1998. *Consilience: The Unity of Knowledge.* Vintage.

Wong, T., et al. 2006. Anxiety among university students during the SARS epidemic in Hong Kong. *Stress and Health* 23, no. 1: 31–35.

Wood, A. 1792–1796. *History and Antiquities of the University of Oxford.*

Woodward, T. 1973. A historical account of the rickettsial diseases with a discussion of the unsolved problems. *Journal of Infectious Disease* 127: 583–594.

Yeager, R. 1996. Military HIV/AIDS Policy in eastern and southern Africa: A seven-country comparison. Occasional paper 1, Civil-Military Alliance to Combat HIV and AIDS.

Youde, J. 2005a. Enter the fourth horseman: Health security and international relations theory. *Whitehead Journal of Diplomacy and International Relations*, March: 193–208.

Youde, J. 2005b. The development of a counter-epistemic community: AIDS, South Africa and international regimes. *International Relations* 19, no. 4: 421–439.

Youde, J. 2007. *AIDS, South Africa, and the Politics of Knowledge.* Ashgate.

Zacher, M., and S. Carvalho. 2001. The international health regulations in historical perspective. In *Plagues and Politics*, ed. A. Price-Smith. Palgrave/Macmillan.

Zartman, I. 1995. *Collapsed States: The Disintegration and restoration of Legitimate Authority.* Lynne Rienner.

Zeigler, R. 2000. *America's Great War: World War I and the American Experience.* Rowman and Littlefield.

Zinsser, H. 1934. *Rats, Lice and History.* Little, Brown.

Index